The Homesteader's
HERBAL COMPANION

THE ULTIMATE GUIDE TO GROWING, PRESERVING, AND USING HERBS

AMY K

Foreword b

GUILFORD,

An imprint of The Rowman & Littlefield Publishing Group, Inc.
4501 Forbes Blvd., Ste. 200
Lanham, MD 20706
www.rowman.com

Distributed by NATIONAL BOOK NETWORK

British Library Cataloguing in Publication Information Available

Library of Congress Cataloging-in-Publication Data

ISBN 978-1-4930-3415-4 (paperback)
ISBN 978-1-4930-3416-1 (e-book)

∞™ The paper used in this publication meets the minimum requirements of American National Standard for Information Sciences—Permanence of Paper for Printed Library Materials, ANSI/NISO Z39.48-1992.

Printed in the United States of America

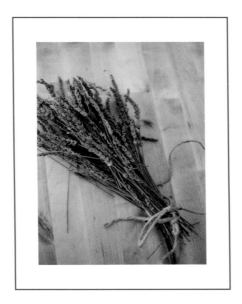

Dedicated to my beautiful husband, son, family, friends,
and blog readers who inspire me to make a difference
for the good, each and every day, no matter what.

CONTENTS

Foreword

When I was an early teenager, my pollen allergies hit me hard enough in the spring and fall that my parents decided it was time to seek medical relief. Living on a farm and growing chickens, I was exposed to dust and pollen levels—especially during hay making season—that were off the charts. I can remember mowing hay with a box of Kleenex perched on the tractor cowling, and when I'd get finished with the field, the white tissues looked like snowballs scattered around.

We went the typical medical procedure route with cortisone. Side effect? "It may erode the cartilage in your nose." Sounds terrific, no? Just what I wanted, to be twenty-five years old and have no cartilage in my nose. When I went to college, away from the farm, I had no problem with the allergies and quit filling the prescription.

After college, I returned to the farm but things seemed better, and by that time our family had drunk more of the naturalist Kool-aid. I just toughed it out spring and fall for several years. The worst was ragweed. Some days in the really tough seasons I would walk around bleary-eyed for a couple of days. I have an extremely high pain and irritation tolerance, so I just powered through the discomfort.

Until we met an herbalist. That changed my life. She introduced us to burdock root. On the farm, we had plenty of burdock, so I went out and dug up a plant, brought the root in to my wife, Teresa, and she followed the recipe: 3 ounces of root, steeped in 4 cups of water for 1 hour. Let sit, and drink 1 cup per meal (4 meals) as a dosage. It was like a miracle. My sinuses cleared up and I returned to the land of the living. Most people, of course, with my level of discomfort, would have been addicted to drugs. I did not feel liberated from the drugs, but I definitely felt liberated from the stranglehold of the allergy. In either case, being liberated is intoxicating.

After reading Amy's book, I now know that this was a decoction (rather than an infusion), and that the dosage matters. In other words, I do not take this every day.

And we don't mess around with the recipe. Teresa faithfully prepares it whenever I come into the house with those telltale allergy sniffles, and within hours I'm in good shape. Once in a while we have to do two rounds to get the final relief, but that's fine. We have plenty of burdock growing in the fields and all it takes is a few minutes in the kitchen.

We had friends who invited us to go camping with them on a lake. They didn't have room in their RV for all of us, so Daniel (my son, who was then about twelve years old) and I elected to sleep in a tent outside. The campground had a common showering facility. About a month after returning home from that excursion, I developed a sore spot in my foot. It got slowly but progressively worse, and we realized I had a plantar wart. Those things can get nasty. Do I need to remind you that I have a high pain threshold? And I'm stubborn as a mule? And I don't like medications?

That plantar wart grew, and I put off doing anything about it until my foot was so sore I limped. Guess who crossed our path about that time? Another herbalist. Suggestion: "Try comfrey." Well goodness, we'd had a bed of comfrey in the garden for forever. We fed it to chickens as a tonic, and rabbits especially like the big hairy leaves. I went out, took a nice succulent leaf, folded it up and put it against the plantar wart, then pulled my sock on over it. It took a little doing to get the hang of keeping it in position, but when I put my shoe back on and stepped on it, the plant juices crushed onto the wart. Within minutes my foot stung mightily . . . and I grinned big time. I knew that if it was stinging, something was happening. I'm a guy of action.

I put a new leaf in every morning for a couple of days, and within a week it was obvious things were changing. The skin around the wart became soft and started pulling away from the wart. I'll try not to gross you out here, but it's really cool how this natural stuff works. It's not immediate, like a knife. It's just gentle and gradual. The built-up layers of skin began peeling off, and within about three weeks, the final big plug of wart just pulled right out. The whole area was surrounded with bright, clean, soft skin that gradually filled in the hole.

I am not an herbalist, but I guarantee you I've become a fan, a disciple, of this kind of gentle, do-it-yourself healing. And I have a deep appreciation for the knowledge that herbalists bring to discussions about what ails us. The overriding word that kept coming to my mind as I read Amy's manuscript was *freedom.* The whole homesteader and DIY movement screams *freedom.*

Freedom from the pharmaceutical companies. Freedom from the medical insurance malaise. Freedom from emergency rooms and hospitals (not completely, of course, but for many of the issues all of us face). The sheer magnitude of being freed up from these costly and debilitating conventions is enormous, and something that should attract every single person, whether you can have your own personal herb garden or not.

The Homesteader's Herbal Companion is both comprehensive and enjoyable. Amy skates perfectly down the middle between science and art. What a joy to have a book like this as a resource for both beginners and old hands. If you've never ventured into the world of herbs, you'll find this book drawing you in and before you know it, I'm sure you'll be dipping your toe in this exciting pool of wisdom. The historical contexts are an enjoyable read by themselves.

From culinary to medicinal, from seat-of-the-pants to technical, and from homestead to urban condominium, this book offers solutions that can free you. Amy captures a wisdom that predates modern pharmacology by eons. We would do well to heed history's successful track record.

Thank you, Amy, for bringing into our lives, our homes, our families such a wealth of freedom. What else could offer this many positives to life with so few negatives? Making herbs ubiquitous in our lives and our kitchens can revolutionize our health and happiness. I encourage all of us to read, enjoy, and then practice this ancient art of wellness freedom.

Joel Salatin

Polyface Farm

Editor, *The Stockman Grass Farmer*

Introduction

I absolutely love herbs. I absolutely love food. I love my family, and they love my herbs and food. See how that works? And I most certainly love living a natural lifestyle. How lovely it is to live a life where nature constantly teaches you new and incredible things each and every day, if you let it. How beautiful it is to watch your child play in the creek behind your house, or walk into the woods and point at the plants that he knows are edible. How pleasing it is to pluck delicate flower heads from chamomile in your garden, or knead rosemary bread on the countertop in the dead of winter.

Herbs are some of my favorite things to grow in my garden, and they go hand in hand with cooking food and living a natural lifestyle, too. The fuzzy leaves on a sage plant, the sweet aroma of thyme infusing the oil in a cast-iron skillet alongside a juicy grass-fed steak—this is just good living. And whether you're on a 100-acre farm, or a backyard homestead in suburbia, incorporating herbs into your food, health products, and livestock routine is absolutely possible to achieve. Learning how to use herbs safely, efficiently, and deliciously is completely attainable.

But before we get too far into this, let me tell you a little more about myself. I grew up in a small Virginia farm town that was literally just a stop sign on a map. In fact, to this day, it's not much different, and I still only live about twenty miles away from where I grew up. My grandparents owned a farm, and still do, and my sister and I loved spending summers there. You'd find us rolling through the fields on a four-wheeler, feeding cows handfuls of grass through the fence line, as if the grass really were greener on the other side. And let's not even talk about calving season, because I could've kissed all those sloppy wet calf noses a thousand times.

It was screen doors, sun tea, fresh cobbler, and nights on the front porch staring at the stars. It was country living at its finest. You could say that it was inevitable for me to choose the farm life. I never quite mastered the farm skills or the lifestyle until my twenties when I began raising my own family. And I certainly never grew up knowing anything about herb gardening or how to use herbs.

I wasn't always conscious of my health. The processed food that I'd put on my plate and the chemical medicine that I'd put in my body—they seemed a normal part of Westernized culture. I never questioned them. In my mind, everything other than what a doctor or grocery store said was normal was "alternative" medicine. So imagine the surprise of some of my friends and family when they saw me pushing fermented foods, offering herbal tinctures and essential oils to them when they were ill, or seeing me out in public wearing muck boots covered in Lord only knows what.

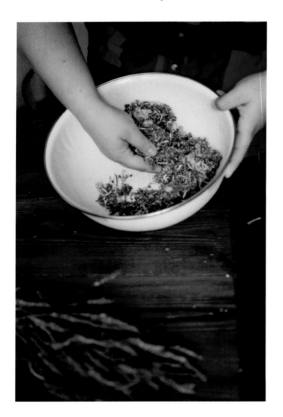

Homesteading—it's not something that I really thought I'd achieve in life. In fact, I haven't quite "achieved" it at all. It's a journey, not necessarily a destination. Life hasn't always gone as planned, but I'm realizing more and more that I'm on the path I'm meant to be on. And oh, the things I have learned and am still learning along the way.

Some of my favorite moments happen in the quiet of the early morning—those moments when I harvest tomatoes and basil from our kitchen garden for the day's lunch, or when I slip a warm, freshly laid chicken egg in my pocket before heading back up to the house after chores, picking leaves of soothing plantain as I go along. There's nothing quite like knowing exactly where your food comes from, and *when* it comes from; it wasn't packed full of chemical ingredients you can't pronounce, and those eggs weren't run through a bleach solution before being packaged.

Nowadays, there's a rooster crowing outside of our bedroom window every single morning. Some days I enjoy it, other days I want to chuck a boot at him before he wakes up my sleeping child. *Just five more minutes of rest, Mr. Rooster. Please, dear Lord, just five more minutes.*

Let's just keep it real here.

There are muddy little boots sitting in the middle of my living room, there's homegrown garlic hanging in my pantry, and I take my coffee a little darker now than I use to . . . and with a dab of fresh butter. My husband, Mark, really enjoys coffee. I think he likes me, too.

While many days are full of homemade meals, homeschool, and beauty, I assure you there is chaos more days of the week than I can count. Let's not even talk about the attitude a farm kid can give you. Amen? But out of chaos comes learning, and how boring would this homesteading life be if everything were always rainbows and unicorns? Out of chaos comes growth, and with growth comes knowledge.

There are often scuffed-up knees, livestock wounds, common colds, and glass in a foot (even after you've told your child to put his shoes back on fifteen times). If mom is down, everyone is down. Thankfully, I now have preventative measures I can take with herbs on my side.

As a wife and mother, my homesteading journey didn't actually begin with animals or a garden. No sir, (or, er, ma'am) it didn't. My personal homesteading journey began with healthcare and herbalism, and wanting to be more self-sufficient in my knowledge of cooking with herbs, using essential oils, and making herbal remedies. I needed to stay healthy, and my son did too. I wanted to make salves, lotions, and soaps. It began with a dream of raising a healthy and happy family which, quite unexpectedly, turned into the warm egg in my pocket and herbs in a garden, and eventually, herbs in my livestock feed, herbs hanging in the coop, and herbs being used throughout the home.

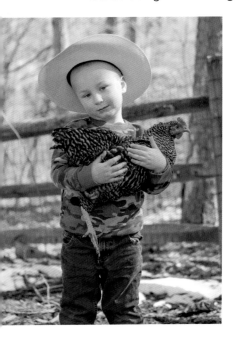

When our son Junior (his real name is Mark) was diagnosed with childhood asthma at the age of twelve months, we turned to a more natural diet and herbal remedies, not just to help treat the issue but in hopes of preventing other issues. During this experience, I not only fell in love with herbalism, I fell in love with farming once again. Realizing that herbalism and farming went hand in hand was liberating. All of it was necessary, every single part of it.

And so we bought a few backyard chickens, rabbits, ducks—and the rest is history. I began growing herbs in containers on my back deck since I didn't have much garden space at the time. But as the years progressed, we created an entire herb garden right in our front yard and then grew everything in a much larger vegetable kitchen garden. All of this took place on half an acre in the middle of a forest sub-division. Grow food, not lawns, right?

Through a combination of modern medicine, herbal remedies, and the grace of God, our son completely outgrew asthma by age six, and I discovered that prevention is the key to living a healthy, natural lifestyle, not just for my family but for our animals and gardens as well.

Nature has given us so many things that we can utilize for our homesteads, but we've lost the skills of knowing how to use them. From creating herbal salves that can heal wounds and soothe coughs, to incorporating herbs into our daily diets to stay healthy and avoid too much salt, to using herbs to keep our livestock healthy, we can learn how to use natural remedies in our homes.

When we learn how to incorporate herbs in our lives, we can eliminate many things within our homes that are filled with chemicals and unnatural ingredients.

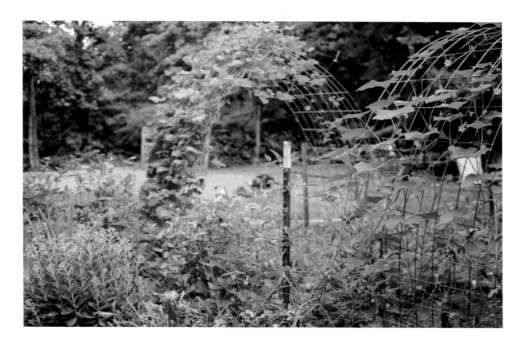

We can create our own household cleaners, and save money while doing so. We can create our own chicken coop and barn cleaners, household air fresheners, cattle fly spray, pest deterrents, and more.

I've so enjoyed learning how to live an herbal lifestyle on our homestead, and I'm excited for the opportunity to share the things that I have learned with you.

I believe that herbalism is an ongoing learning experience.

I also believe that, initially, herbalism can be overwhelming and scary. That's why I'll start off with some of the top herbs that anyone can use. I dislike having too many options. Just tell me what I need, sister, and I'm good to go!

You don't need two hundred different herbs in your garden for four different ailments—you'll never use them all. I'll teach you what to grow in your garden *and* which wild herbs to forage. And, when necessary, there are a lot of great options from which you can outsource herbs instead of growing them yourself.

In this book, you'll learn all about the basics of herbalism: how to start your herb garden; tips on growing herbs, cooking with herbs, incorporating herbs into your

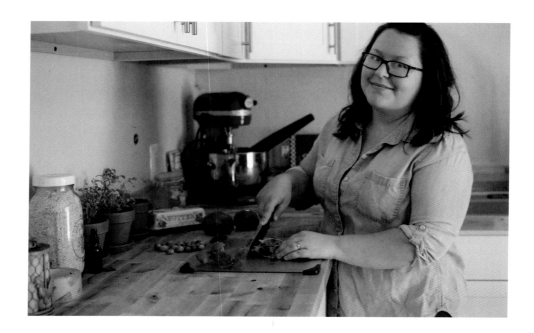

daily routine, making and using herbal products (like salves, tinctures, and essential oils); and how to incorporate herbs in and around your home, outbuildings, and barns, and with your livestock. You'll learn about using and preserving herbs, and so much more.

While I'm not a doctor, certified practitioner, or professional chef, I am a mom, wife, and herbalist who longs for a better lifestyle for my family. And as we all know, moms and wives can research better than anyone, especially when it comes to their family's safety! And more than anything, ***I'm living it, and it works.***

Herbalism should be exciting. And that's why I wrote this book.

This is the book I wish I could have referenced when I first started my journey.

This is the book that I hope encourages you along your own.

Happy herbing!

Amy

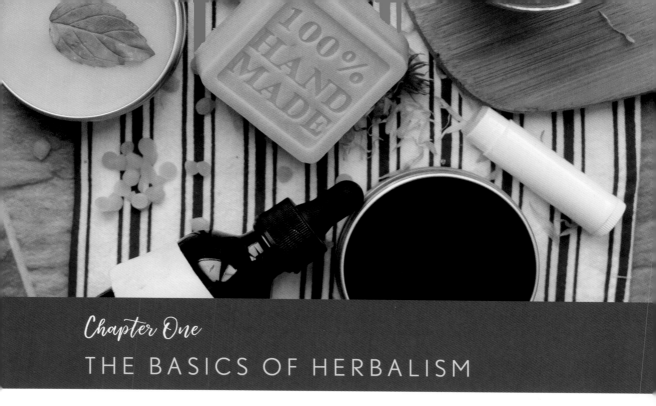

Chapter One

THE BASICS OF HERBALISM

Before the advent of modern medicine, herbalism was the one and only way to treat your family and prevent illness. We used herbs to season foods that we prepared for our families. We used them during rituals and burials. We used them as offerings, teas, incense, and so much more.

On a farm, you knew how to take care of yourself, because the nearest doctor wasn't often . . . well . . . near. Our great-grandparents cooked with herbs, farmed with herbs, and treated their illnesses with herbs. More than anything, they knew *how* to do this.

Our ancestors could walk right out the back door and tell us what this plant or that plant was. They could tell us why dandelions were good for your liver and kidneys, not just a pest weed. They could pick lavender from the garden and tell you how well it works for burns and wounds, and even to help them or their babies relax. They ate their meals with herbs and spices that had healing properties— things that we think are simply culinary additions in today's world. Back then, herbs

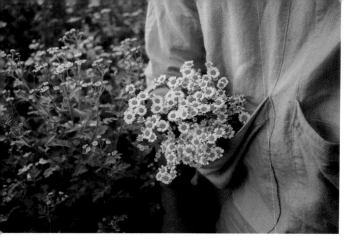

had great purpose when propagated in a natural way, in the garden, encouraged by sunshine and the hands of an enthusiastic caretaker.

In modern society, most of the herbs we grow originate from the Middle East, Europe, and the Mediterranean. Thankfully, many of the plants have adapted to our differing climates across the world over the centuries, although some herbs, like basil and cilantro, still require special care.

Homesteaders today are on a mission to get back to their roots and regain knowledge that has dwindled for generations. We cook with herbs that we've grown in our gardens. We make salves, soaps, and lotions for our bodies. We learn about essential oils, which are herbs in one of their more potent forms. And we're even learning how to utilize herbs with our livestock, in our pastures, and in our household cleaners.

HERBALISM HISTORY

Until the Middle Ages, herbs were used by ancient cultures for a variety of purposes. When people started to assume that disease and illness were punishments from God, they tossed herbalism and natural healing aside. Thankfully, many monks opened their doors to those who wanted to continue their herbalist educations and to those who were already knowledgeable. Many monasteries grew beautiful herb gardens in their courtyards. They offered their services and herbal remedies to those in need.

Fast-forward to the eighteenth and nineteenth centuries, when scientific discoveries on the causes of diseases and how they are transmitted were at the forefront of modern medicine. We made major strides in sanitation and vaccinations to decrease communicable diseases. Unfortunately, the notion that all disease could be completely eradicated led to the decline in the practice of herbalism as preventative medicine.

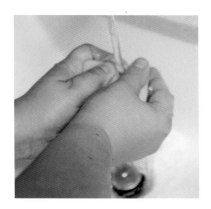

The decrease in herbalism and skilled natural medicine was rapid, and unfortunately, we are still paying for it today. Not even a year after the discovery of antibiotics, we became an antibiotic-resistant people. And now, we are quickly nearing the end of the antibiotic era. Antibiotics are used in our livestock feeds, injected into commercial meat animals for faster food production, slathered on wounds through antibiotic ointments, and overused and abused by many.

This is why many people, especially homesteaders, are turning back to herbalism, not just to heal, but to live a more natural lifestyle. And that's not just for our bodies, but for our animals and food as well. We are turning away from the overuse of antibiotics and other unnatural product additives. And we know that in order for this herbalism thing to work in a modern society, we must remaster the practice before we reach the post-antibiotic era.

It's time to take back our homes, our health, our food, and our lives.

WHAT ARE HERBS?

So first, the age-old question, *what are herbs*? Once you understand this, you'll be set, my friend! Then, and only then, can we get to the fun stuff!

Believe it or not, there are many people who just think of herbs as beautiful plants to cook with. And while you can absolutely cook with them—and I'll show you how in this book—they are so much more useful in so many ways.

Herbs are plants used for food, flavoring, medicine, or fragrances. They are used for their savory, medicinal, or aromatic properties. Herbs can be used in cooking, through aromatics, and through herbal medicine. They can also be used to provide everyday nutritional balance.

HERBALISM SAFETY

This is the part where I tell you not to kill yourself with herbs. Seriously, **read this section.** Just do it, because I don't ever want to say, "I told you so."

Whether you are using herbs in a tincture or using them with essential oils, there really are some safety precautions you should take. It's not to deter you from using them, it's simply to encourage you to use the smarts you were blessed with. Also, there's no sense in using herbs if you aren't going to use them properly, because they plumb won't work.

Let me first say that if you're just using herbs to cook, there aren't too many precautions you need to take unless you're allergic to herbs of a certain plant family. There's a big difference between the amount of an herb you cook with, and the amount of an herb you'd take medicinally. It's essential to know the difference between medicinal and tonic herbs (which I'll explain in the following pages), and to know that you should use caution if you have a health condition, are on medications, are pregnant or nursing, and before using them with your children or the elderly.

Ultimately, I want you to feel confident using herbs on even your smallest child, because I know that when you want something to work, you want to understand exactly how it works without fear of hurting your family or livestock.

MEDICINAL VERSUS TONIC HERBS

Whether you're using them for medicine or just to make a simple lotion, you need to know how to safely use herbs. Just as with antibiotics, too much of a good thing can be a bad thing in herbalism. It's extremely important to know that there are two different classes of herbs when it comes to healing and use in everyday life: **medicinal herbs** and **tonic herbs.**

Medicinal Herbs are herbs that typically have a strong chemistry. Medicinal herbs are generally not to be consumed in large doses unless directed by your physician, and can be harmful to the body if not taken properly. When using medicinal herbs, you typically take specific dosages (sometimes large amounts) for two weeks at a time, and then take a break before starting again. These herbs operate with our bodies in specific ways to treat specific ailments. They can be considered toxic if not taken properly or in too large a dosage. However, the toxicity of most of these herbs occurs with such high doses that we would never even think of dosing ourselves at that level.

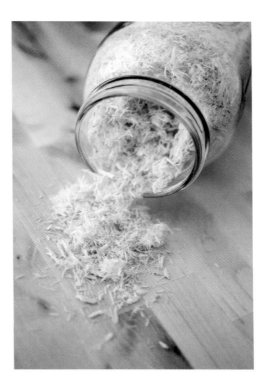

Medicinal herbs can be used in smaller amounts in cooking. Take garlic, for example. Like me, you probably cook with it almost daily. But when taken in large doses, garlic can be a powerful medicinal herb in the body and can be toxic when taken in excess (20 grams or more a day). Don't worry, however, about adding that much to Sunday night's homemade pasta dinner!

Know what you need!

A man once asked me why he was having heart flutterings while taking echinacea to boost his immunity. When I asked him how long and how much he had been taking, I was shocked to find out that he took a high dosage supplement every single day because a friend had told him to take it. He was having heart flutterings because his body didn't need the echinacea, and because he'd been taking too much of it for an extended amount of time. It's important to know this when diving into the medicinal herb field.

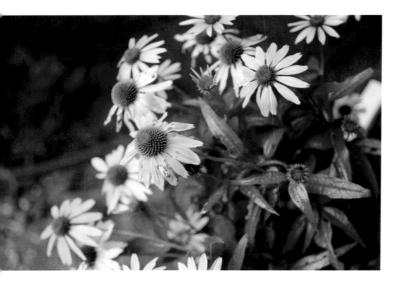

Similarly, herbs like comfrey, which many homesteaders grow in their gardens, have been proven time and time again to cause toxicity (especially of the liver) when ingested in large amounts. It's always best to research dosing from a reliable source before using your herbs. Remember, just because someone says it's true, doesn't mean that it is.

Slow and steady wins the race, and taking the time to know your stuff really pays off in the end. Examples of medicinal herbs are echinacea, garlic, comfrey, arnica (never to be ingested), and holy basil.

Tonic Herbs are herbs that are for general usage and can be consumed in large amounts without fear of toxicity. However, I still caution people not to consume them in extra-large dosages. They have a generalized health effect on many areas of the body or the whole body in general rather than targeting a specific ailment like medicinal herbs do. Low in toxicity but high in benefits, these herbs are given for general ailments or for overall health and are also great for cooking and regular consumption. Some examples of tonic herbs are parsley, cilantro, and ginger.

No matter what type of herb you use, whether medicinal or tonic, **all herbs in their natural state have the ability to cause irritation if not taken properly,** or if you have an allergy to them. With that said, you've more than likely been using herbs like thyme, basil, garlic, turmeric, and rosemary in your cooking for years. If these haven't bothered you, keep using them. It is the actual extraction in a tea, tincture, salve, or syrup that may cause adverse reactions.

Herbs can be used to make hot water infusions (or teas), tinctures, syrups, poultices, macerates, infused oils, salves, creams, powders, or essential oils . . . the list goes on. In this book, you'll learn about several of these forms, and how and when to use them.

Most of the parts of an herb—such as the flowers, leaves, seeds, and roots—can be used, but they may have

Don't eat it . . .

Not all herbs can be, or should be, ingested. For example, arnica is an herb we use to heal pain from the outside in, but it should never be ingested for healing from the inside out. Or at least, not without medical supervision. In other words, don't eat it! Do your research. Just because you can use something externally doesn't mean it should be used internally.

different benefits. For example, the root of the echinacea plant is typically harvested and turned into a tincture for a more powerful medicinal option. But the leaves can be harvested, dried, and given to livestock or crushed into teas for a lesser medicinal effect. How the medicinal property of the herb is extracted will determine your dosage and what you'll use it for.

SAFE DOSAGES

It's important to know the difference between what's right for daily intake and medicinal intake dosages. This isn't something you'll ever know off the top of your head unless you use an herb often. If an herb isn't working medicinally for you, you might have the dosage too low, and you should consult a certified herbalist or holistic doctor, or up your dosage in extremely small increments. Dosing as a preventative measure versus dosing as a medicinal healing agent are two completely different things and you'll learn about that in just a moment.

The key to dosage is to remember that there's a balancing act between too little, too much, and just the right amount. Knowing the exact amount that's in

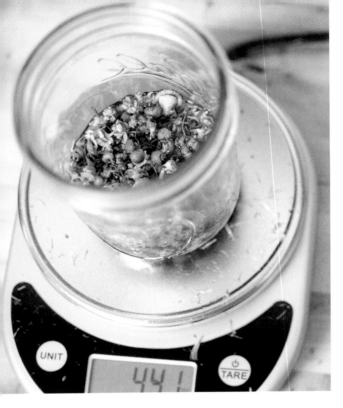

an herbal remedy for your family or livestock is important (this is where our ratio comes in later in the book), and is the difference between healing, not working at all, or toxicity. For this reason, you should always weigh your herbs instead of measuring by cup or by handfuls. A half-pound of oregano looks a whole lot different than a half-pound of calendula. In fact, the calendula will most likely look like three times the amount of oregano, and yet, it's the same exact amount. Measuring by weight is extremely important. We'll talk about this more in chapter 6.

It's also important to understand that the potency of an herb in a hot water tea is not the same potency as an herb that's been extracted in a tincture. Either way, the general rule of thumb for dosing is typically based on the weight of a 150-pound adult, and for children, you simply need to go by weight and age from there (see box). You can think of dosing by age or by weight.

GENERAL ADULT DOSAGE AMOUNTS
TINCTURE: 30 drops or 1 eyedropper (1-ounce bottle), 1–3 times a day
SYRUP: 1–2 tsp a day for preventative, 1–3 tbsp every 3 hours to heal
ESSENTIAL OIL: 2–3 drops topically, 1–3 drops in capsule internally
TEA: 1–3 tsp dried herbal tea or herb in 8 ounces of water

Accounting for the right dosage

Here are some rules to consider, taken from PhD candidate Jessie Hawkins of The Vintage Remedies Learning Center.

If we're trying to get the dosage for a five-year-old child by weight and by age:

AUSBERGER'S RULE: Convert the **weight** to kilograms (kg), rounding to a whole number. Multiply it by 1.5. Add 10 to arrive at the percentage of the adult dose to use. Example: 18 x 1.5 = 27; 27 + 10 = 37, so the five-year-old's dose would be slightly over one-third of the adult dose or 1.85 milliliters (mL).

CLARK'S RULE: Convert the **weight** to kg, rounding to a whole number. Divide that number by 67. Multiply the sum by the adult dose to obtain the child's dose. Example: 40 pounds (lbs) = approximately 18 kg; 18 ÷ 67 = 0.269; 0.269 × 5 = 1.345 or 1.34 mL.

FRIED'S RULE: While the other rules are suitable for older children, **this one is ideal for infants and very young children.** Begin with the child's **age in months.** Divide by 150, then multiply by the adult dose to arrive at the child's dose. Our example would be: 10 months ÷ 150 = 0.067; 0.067 × 5 = 0.335 or 0.34 mL.

YOUNG'S RULE: Multiply child's age to adult dose. Divide that product by child's age plus 12. Example: 5 (years) × 5 (mL) = 25; Divide by (5 (years) + 12) = 25 ÷ 17 = 1.47 mL.

Younger children are best dosed by weight. Older children and adults are best dosed by age. But when in doubt, weight is always best to go by. When dosing an infant, it's best to allow that infant to receive herbal care through mother's milk; otherwise, weight dosing is best.

Essential oils and liquid extracts are dosed by drops and dropperfuls, but of course it is all dependent upon the type of oil and extract.

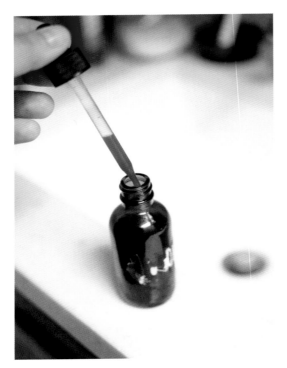

All of this information is readily available to you online through most state college research documents and through trusted herbal schools. Simply plug in your herb name and the recommended dosage, and you'll receive the recommended scientific dosage of the herb. However, I'd highly suggest that if you're serious about the medicinal side of herbalism, you should consider taking an online course through a reputable instructor, which you can find in the resources section of this book.

Of course, when using herbs simply to season food, these rules don't typically apply. All good things in moderation! And when in doubt, ask a holistic professional.

YOUR HEALTH BEFORE HERBS

If you've gotten this far, I applaud you. You actually heeded my warning and you get a gold star! Or a lavender one . . . whichever. Hopefully, you now have a new-found appreciation for herbs after reading this section.

For those who suffer from ailments such as leaky gut syndrome, allergies, diabetes, chronic migraines, and autoimmune diseases, there are a few considerations to make before incorporating herbs in our daily health practices.

If you have skin allergies, herbs may irritate your already inflamed skin. Make sure you're using the proper ones. And make sure you don't have a ragweed allergy, as some of the very herbs that can heal skin irritations come from the ragweed family. Imagine the combination of itchy skin, and slathering more itchiness on top of it!

If you have a chronic illness, before you take any type of herb dosage beyond culinary seasoning, you really should check with your doctor first, or at least do extensive research through herbal publications that strictly focus on the medicinal properties of herbs. For example, if you have epilepsy or a condition that causes seizures, then you should stay away from herbs that could induce seizures (or interact with seizure medications). If you have rheumatoid arthritis, then you should stay away from most immune-stimulating herbs . . . and so on.

If you have leaky gut syndrome, some herbs, like cayenne, might cause irritation.

In all things, be safe! Being cautious is really the best way to approach herbalism. But don't be scared—just be smart about it!

HERB SAFETY FOR CHILDREN AND THE ELDERLY

Young children and the elderly are more susceptible to issues and irritation when it comes to using herbs (whether it's straight herbs or essential oils). For example, for children under the age of eighteen months, it's recommended to avoid the use of essential oils like peppermint and eucalyptus because these can slow their breathing if given in high dosages on the skin. It's similar with the elderly. Many elderly people are on medications,

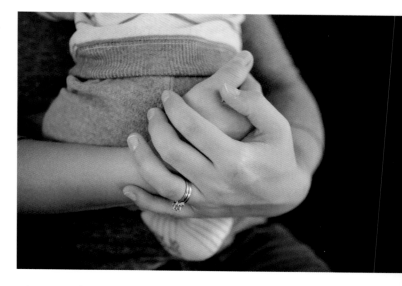

and herbs can be powerful enough to interfere with them. However, they can be greatly beneficial as well.

Use extra caution when giving herbs (in all forms) to Junior and Grammie. And when in doubt, ask a professional. **But don't let that deter you from expanding your own knowledge and trying alternative herbs.** If one herb can't be used, there are usually other herbs and herbal remedies that can be substituted that have a similar effect.

Use with caution
Some herbs to use with caution on children and the elderly:

Peppermint	Black Cohosh	Wormwood
Eucalyptus	Feverfew	Borage
Goldenseal	Comfrey	

HERBS TO AVOID DURING PREGNANCY

Most of us female homesteaders just love knowing there's a future mini-farmhand growing in our bellies. And some of us want to start our herbal journey when we're expanding and growing our family.

While this is an exceptional way to begin your herbal lifestyle, there are some herbs you should avoid during pregnancy when taken in medicinal doses. Now, there are many herbs that you can still use in cooking, but taking them in high medicinal doses is an absolute no-no. See the difference here? It's important to know the difference between daily, culinary, and medicinal intake.

As long as you are using them in culinary food intake, not medicinal intake, herbs like garlic, turmeric, rosemary, sage, and ginger are all okay. Taken in high medicinal dosages, they are not recommended.

There are most certainly more to name, but they are typically uncommon for most homesteaders to grow or use. Our goal is to not be overrun with so many hundreds of different herbs that we forget how to use them appropriately.

Use with caution
Herbs to avoid in high doses during pregnancy:

Roman Chamomile	Wormwood	Aloe
Goldenseal	Comfrey	Sage
Passion Flower	Borage	Peppermint
Yarrow	Red Clover	Thyme
Mugwort	Oregano	

HERBS TO AVOID WITH ANIMALS

There are some herbs you just simply want to avoid with animals, or be very cautious when using. Again, keep in mind we're talking about medicinal dosages here. A little bit of garlic in the chickens' feed isn't going to have detrimental effects, just like putting tea tree essential oil on a dog's wound most likely won't cause issues. That said, the right dosage is extremely important with the following herbs when using them around animals.

Use with caution
Herbs to use with caution with your pets and livestock:

Tea Tree Essential Oil	St. John's Wort	Cohosh (Black or Blue)
Comfrey	Borage	Black Walnut Hulls
Garlic	Goldenseal	

This isn't to say that you can't give these herbs to your animals, but use caution when doing so. Make sure you aren't throwing an entire basket of comfrey in the barnyard and you'll be good to go.

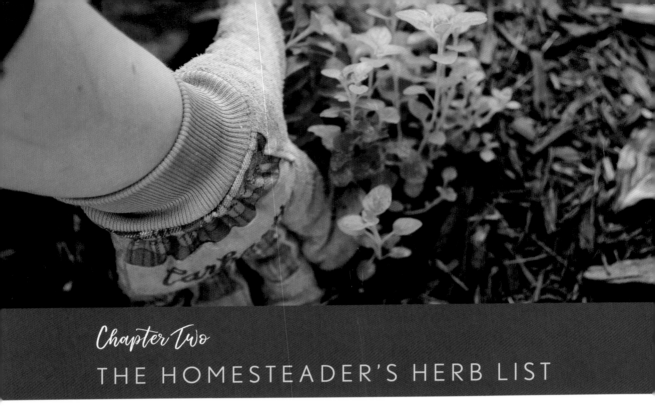

Chapter Two

THE HOMESTEADER'S HERB LIST

Starting an herb garden can be intimidating. I mean, what on earth do you put in that thing? Well, herbs of course. But where would one even begin to whittle down what kinds of herbs to plant? Do they need extra fertilizer? Do they need special treatment? Will I kill them? Will I kill my family? Do I need two hundred herbs in order to accomplish everything I want to?

Calm down there. You've got this. Just take a few deep breaths.

Well, starting an herb garden is simple really. And no, you won't hurt anyone in the process. I promise. A little fertile soil, a little water, a good amount of sunlight—this is just good ol' basic elementary science, my friend. And really, truly, that's all *most* herbs need.

CHOOSING FIVE HERBS FOR YOUR GARDEN

The easiest way to begin your herb garden is to choose five herbs that best suit your homestead needs. My initial list looked something like this:

respiratory

seasonal allergies

common cold and flu

wounds

pretty things

Yes, "pretty things" was definitely on my list. I wanted some herbs just for their aromatic benefits, like lavender, and to be pretty, too. I failed miserably at lavender all three times I grew it the first year, but I continued to try!

As our homesteading journey went on, so did my needs. My list now looks a lot like this:

respiratory

common cold and flu

nausea

leaky gut

boils and cysts

chicken health

bleeding

toothache

broken bones

deep wounds

high blood pressure

migraines

overall livestock health

parasite eradication

culinary uses

and so much more

Wow, what a list, right?

While this list looks overwhelming, luckily I only need a few herbs to treat many issues!

As I dove further into homesteading, I found that when the simple things worked, I wanted more. I didn't just want to only grow for the common cold, I wanted to grow for everything that we might need and to preserve it for long periods of time. I wanted to create things with my herbs too: household products, salves, and lotions. I wanted to cook amazing meals that would be remembered by family. I wanted to live a truly herbal lifestyle.

So **how do you figure out what to grow in your herb garden?** While it can be very overwhelming, it doesn't have to be. *You don't actually have to grow everything.* There are incredible herbal resources online from which you can purchase dried herbs. However, there is a great way to begin your herb garden, and it takes the overwhelming part out of the equation!

To begin, **choose the top five herbs you want to grow the first year you begin this adventure.** You can have five herbs that are strictly culinary in one section, five that are strictly medicinal in another, and so on. Or, you can just start out with five herbs total. Whichever is easiest for you. The key is to choose the things that your homestead and family need the most. Get to know those few herbs the first year, top to bottom. Then the following year (or once you've learned all there is to know about those herbs), add more.

Maybe you deal with respiratory issues, in which case you'd want to grow or forage for yarrow. Maybe your spouse or your mother deals with chronic migraines, in which case feverfew would be a good remedy. You want herbs to add to your livestock feed? Well then, you'll need thyme, oregano, and garlic. That's five herbs right there, and I'm sure you could think of at least ten more you might need. The important thing to remember is to start small your first year so that you don't overwhelm yourself. Take your time to really dive into the attributes of these herbs. If you feel like you can take on more (I most certainly did), then jump right in. You can have a section for medicinal herbs, a separate section for culinary herbs, and again, a separate section for whatever it is you wish. Many homesteaders separate

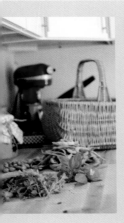

Sample Beginner's Herb Garden

CULINARY HERBS:	MEDICINAL HERBS:	WILD HERBS:
Thyme	Lavender	Yarrow
Oregano	Peppermint	Feverfew
Basil	Chamomile	Elderberry
Rosemary	Echinacea	Red Clover
Garlic	Calendula	Plantain

their herb gardens into sections so they're easier to maintain, but you'll find that many of your culinary herbs overlap with your medicinal ones.

As homesteading often leads to a simpler lifestyle, remember to keep this simple. You don't need hundreds and hundreds of herbs, because you'll find the herbs you do grow have multiple benefits. I repeat, you don't need all the herbs. Step away from the herbs.

You may find that once you've mastered this beginner's list, you might not need anything else at your homestead. But if you do, then I have another great list for you.

THE HOMESTEADER'S HERB LIST

Here's a list of my top homestead herbs, both medicinal and culinary, how we use them, and what they can be used for. There are several wild herbs that I'll add to this list later in the book. For this section, I'll just talk about herbs that I typically grow in my garden or herbs that I buy and use regularly on our homestead. For the wild herbs section, I'll talk about herbs that grow naturally in the wild in most parts of the country, and also herbs that you can grow in a garden bed. You may see a crossover in some of these herb sections because some wild herbs aren't readily available in some regions.

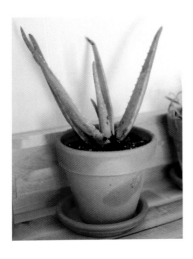

Aloe Plant

Botanical Name: *Aloe vera*

Family: Liliaceae

Common Name(s): aloe, Barbadoes aloe

Perennial growth

Parts used: leaves

Uses: soothes irritated or burned skin, antibacterial, antifungal, anti-inflammatory

Harvest: Break off leaves at the base of the plant, taking outer leaves first. Only harvest as needed. Store unused portion in refrigerator. Aloe is best grown indoors in cooler climates, although gardeners in warm southern climates can easily grow this plant outdoors. I'm located in Virginia, and I've only ever grown it as an indoor plant. It does great in a sunny window!

History: Aloe has traditionally been used as a skin-soothing herb throughout the ages. Many people even ingest the viscous portion of the plant to soothe digestive issues. You can find aloe in skin care products and as straight aloe gel to heal minor burns or sunburned skin. It moisturizes the skin, dry scalp, and damaged hair while inducing healing. Aloe can also be ingested under certain circumstances. It has been proven to help people with irritable bowel syndrome (IBS) when drinking 30 milliliters (mL) twice a day. It has also been used to treat stomach ulcers.

How We Use It: We use it in the same way most people would. I keep an aloe plant on hand for those times when I burn myself in the kitchen, when someone burns themselves on an engine, or when we need it for various other skin irritants. It also goes great in a salve with calendula.

Safety and Dosage: Do not ingest aloe if pregnant or nursing. Do not take high doses of aloe. Do not use for an extended period of time. Do not ingest aloe if you have diabetes or are on laxative medications. It is not suggested that you try to harvest the viscous portion of the plant yourself for *internal* use. You can do so for external use. Do not take more than 200 mg each day for longer than four weeks.

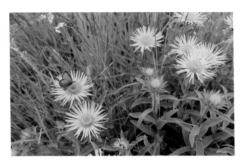

Arnica

Botanical Name: *Arnica montana*

Family: Asteraceae

Common Name(s): leopard's bane, mountain tobacco, mountain arnica

Perennial growth

Parts used: flowers, root

Uses: induces perspiration, heals wounds, reduces aches, pains, bruises, sprains, inflammation, and overexerted muscles

Harvest: Cut flowers when in bloom in the early morning.

History: Arnica has long been used for external medicine throughout Europe and North America. Native Americans made healing ointments with the native species of arnica for wounds and strained muscles. In modern society, arnica is most popularly used in the same way—for relaxing stiff muscles, treating wounds, healing sprains and bruises, and aiding inflamed skin.

How We Use It: My favorite way to use arnica is in a salve, lotion, or balm. This is a great way to safely use its healing properties. You can learn how to make these products throughout the book. Use the products on your loved ones and on your animals.

Safety and Dosage: Arnica is an herb that should never be taken internally, as it can be extremely toxic—use arnica externally only. Oils, balms, salves, and lotions should only contain 10 to 15 percent arnica. Arnica is never to be applied to open wounds or broken skin. If you have extremely sensitive skin, you may have an adverse reaction. If so, discontinue use.

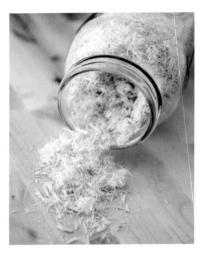

Astragalus

Botanical Name: *Astragalus membranaceus*

Family: Fabaceae

Common Name(s): membranous milkvetch, huang-qi

Perennial growth

Parts used: roots

Uses: immune support, helps body adapt to stress, antibacterial, antiviral, reduces the common cold and flu, increases white blood cell count, anti-inflammatory, protects cardiovascular system

Harvest: The root can be harvested after three to four years of growth.

History: Astragalus has a deep history in Chinese medicine, much like ginseng. It has been traditionally used for over five thousand years to help boost the immune system and cure many common ailments.

How We Use It: Astragalus is the new favorite herb in the Fewell home. Combined with elderberry, it truly is a powerhouse herb remedy that helps boost immunity and practically cures the common cold. It's also a great preventative, especially when taken before you go out to germ-breeding grounds like grocery stores, amusement parks, holiday events, and playgrounds. We also use it in our livestock tinctures.

Safety and Dosage: A 1:5 tincture ratio can be taken three times a day, 30 drops per dose. It can be taken in a syrup of 1–2 teaspoons (tsp) to prevent illness and common cold. Or take in an elderberry syrup at the elderberry dosage (see recipe on page 127). There are no known safety precautions with this herb, and it is considered safe for general usage.

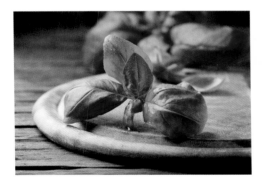

Basil

Botanical Name: *Ocimum basilicum*

Family: Lamiaceae

Common Name(s): sweet basil, garden basil, common basil

Annual growth

Parts used: leaves

Uses: rich in antioxidants, mood enhancer, anti-inflammatory, antidepressant, headache aid, digestive issues, regulates gut flora, supports the immune system

Harvest: Harvest basil leaves throughout the season, taking just the tops off, or cutting down to the newest set of small leaves. This ensures that you will get basil all season long.

History: Basil has always been a luxurious herb and is often associated with Italian food and fine dining. It is originally native to India but has made its way all around the world. Basil is rich in antioxidants, uplifts mood, aids in depression, and brings mental clarity, all by its scent alone. It aids the body as an anti-inflammatory, which means we just love eating it all the time for this very reason! Basil helps the body adjust to changes and stress, and herbalists encourage people to eat it often during those times to aid in emotional support and inflammation in the body.

How We Use It: We eat it, plain and simple. I *love* basil, which is funny, because I *hated* basil until I began growing it myself. Funny how that seems to work. We use it in pesto, on pizza, in pasta sauce, on tomatoes with feta. Sweet goodness, the possibilities are endless with summertime basil! Basil is also great as an "eat-your-medicine" type of herb. If I know my family is going through a stressful time or is in need of a boost, I make a meal with lots and lots of basil. Because basil is good like that.

Safety and Dosage: There are no known precautions, however, pregnant women should limit their use of basil to culinary use only. Typical dose of dried basil is 800 mg per day.

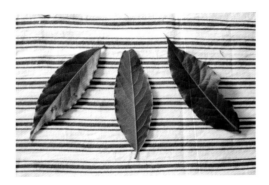

Bay Leaf

Botanical Name: *Laurus nobilis*

Family: Lauraceae

Common Name(s): bay laurel, sweet bay, true bay

Perennial growth

Parts used: leaves

Uses: antibacterial, antioxidant, antifungal, lowers blood sugar, aids digestion, soothes digestive tract, rheumatism/arthritis

Harvest: Harvest leaves throughout the season.

History: The bay leaf is sprinkled throughout history. From mystic folklore to Roman emperors, everyone has used bay leaf. It was an herb of glory and reward, it was considered romantic, and it was widely used to ease menstruation, heal wounds, and take away rheumatism. Bay leaf is a fabulous herb to cook with and is most often found in dishes that include chicken. This herb is best grown in warm climates. It can be grown in less warm climates but should be brought indoors during the cold months.

How We Use It: I love cooking with bay leaf. It is one of the main herbs in many of my chicken dishes, in my chicken stock, and in my chicken noodle soup. It smells fabulous, and you can also find it in a citrus and cinnamon potpourri that I leave sitting in my wood stove humidifier in the winter.

Safety and Dosage: There are no known safety precautions with this herb. Tinctures of a 1:5 ratio can be taken up to three times per day, 30 drops each time.

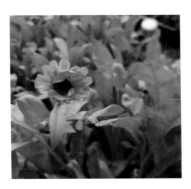

Calendula

Botanical Name: *Calendula officinalis*

Family: Asteraceae

Common Name(s): pot marigold, marigold, garden marigold

Annual growth

Parts used: flowers

Uses: anti-inflammatory, stimulates wound healing, gastrointestinal issues

Harvest: Harvest flower heads at maturity, dry out before using.

History: The ancient Romans are most known for growing calendula, and they even gave it its name. However, it didn't come into major medicinal use until later in history. Calendula has been used for toothaches, headaches, red eyes, fevers, wound healing, and skin soothing. It is also still used as a natural dye. Today, we use calendula to soothe, bring relief from inflammation, speed up wound healing, and bring relief to irritated skin.

How We Use It: I think I put calendula in just about every salve I make. I'm kidding—kind of. But it truly has incredible benefits for the skin and your body. We have seen major skin irritations, bee stings, and other "ouchies" healed by calendula salves! It can also be safely used on livestock. Calendula is in my pantry 24/7!

Safety and Dosage: There are not any known conditions that would prohibit people from using calendula, unless they are allergic to plants in the ragweed family. Obviously its use should be discontinued if a skin reaction occurs, but this is very rare. Salves and creams should offer an herbal content of at least 5 percent. We generally apply calendula topically and externally.

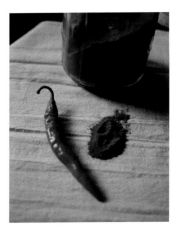

Cayenne (capsicum)

Botanical Name: *Capsicum annuum*

Family: Solanaceae

Common Name(s): cayenne, chili pepper

Annual growth (perennial growth in warmer zones)

Parts used: fruits, dried and powdered

Uses: digestive aid, stimulant, muscle spasm and pain reducer, arthritis, antibacterial, counter-irritant

Harvest: Harvest peppers when mature, then dehydrate (or hang to dry) and turn into a powder.

History: People often don't think that cayenne pepper is an herb, but we forget than an herb is any plant we use for its medicinal or aromatic purposes. Cayenne was first introduced to Europe when Christopher Columbus returned from the Americas. We saw cayenne appear in our history books back in 1493, and in the sixteenth century, cayenne pepper really began to be noticed for its medicinal and culinary properties. Cayenne peppers have more vitamin C content than oranges, and a large amount of vitamin A. Cayenne gets its heat and medicinal properties from capsaicin, which is a component in the pepper. Because of this, we use cayenne sparingly for muscle pains, back pain, and arthritis, in creams, poultices, or salves.

How We Use It: You can find a pain-reducing salve in this book that we use on ourselves when we need extra pain reduction on sore muscles and joints (see page 152).

Safety and Dosage: Cayenne can cause skin irritation. It's probably best not to use it on children. A little bit truly does go a long way. Be sure to wash hands thoroughly after using.

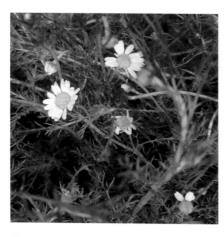

Chamomile

Botanical Name: *Matricaria recutita*

Family: Asteraceae

Common Name(s): German chamomile

Annual growth

Parts used: flowers, entire plant

Uses: anti-inflammatory, antispasmodic, mild sedative, digestive aid, helps heal mucous membranes

Harvest: Harvest your flower tops in the early morning hours when the petals begin to fall back. Store in an airtight container after drying thoroughly.

History: There are two main types of chamomile—Roman chamomile and German chamomile. The entire chamomile family is medicinally beneficial in similar ways. There are simply different characteristics for each. For example, the flower petals of German chamomile are squarer, whereas the petals of Roman chamomile are a bit more wispy and pointed. Roman chamomile is a perennial, while German chamomile is more often an annual, unless it self-seeds. For centuries, the chamomile family has been used for its gentle healing properties. Chamomile is most commonly used as a digestive aid and for its anti-inflammatory properties. It is also known to calm the nervous system. It can be used in many different ways—infused in a tea or even used in a salve. The volatile oils in chamomile help heal inflammation of the skin and mucous membranes. Chamomile also helps with indigestion and inflammation of the digestive tract. Used topically, it makes a great salve or balm for diaper rash, eczema, psoriasis, wounds, and bruises. Chamomile promotes a restful sleep and is fabulous for adults and children who need help relaxing before bedtime. Chamomile has an apple-like fragrance, and can bring a sense of calm to any room.

How We Use It: I love using chamomile in salves, lotions, balms, and infused oils. Chamomile tea is also a must for tummy troubles and restless nights in our household. Make a fabulous anti-inflammatory salve out of chamomile, calendula, and arnica for your family and animals.

Safety and Dosage: If you are allergic to ragweed or any of the plants in the ragweed family, you may have an allergic reaction to chamomile. Otherwise, no other dangers are known for this herb. Steep 2–3 teaspoons of crushed dried chamomile flower tops in a cup of hot water to create a tea. Chamomile is best used externally through an herbal product, or internally through a tea or infusion rather than a tincture; however, it can be blended with other herbs in a tincture.

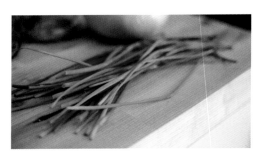

Chives

Botanical Name:
Allium Schoenoprasum

Family: Liliaceae

Perennial growth

Parts used: scapes and flowers

Uses: mostly culinary, aides in digestion, may be helpful with anemia

Harvest: Cut chive scapes before they blossom for a robust taste in culinary dishes. Leave about two inches in sections, not taking the entire clump of chives, if you want the plant to continue growing. Use chives immediately or dehydrate them for later use. Flowers can be snipped and eaten fresh in salads and other dishes.

History: Chives have a sweet, oniony taste, and are best eaten when fresh. These are perfect for the person who doesn't like the bitterness of regular onions and just wants a hint of flavor. Like most herbs, we've seen chives in dishes across the world for thousands of years, dating back to the ancient Greeks and Chinese. Chives are often used in dishes with vegetables from the garden. The colonists brought chives to America, and we've been in love with them ever since. Our ancestors believed that chives could keep diseases and evil spirits away, but science and real life have shown us otherwise. While chives are tasty, they don't have much medicinal benefit, but they might keep away vampires!

How We Use It: Because chives really lack in the medicinal category, I only use chives in culinary dishes. Chives are also wonderful as a companion plant in the garden, helping deter pests from other plants. And, let's face it, they're just beautiful to look at!

Safety and Dosage: While chives do hold some medicinal value, you would have to eat a *lot* of them in order to receive any of those benefits. However, it would also cost you an upset and painful stomach from overeating them. Stick to the culinary uses and there are no safety precautions necessary.

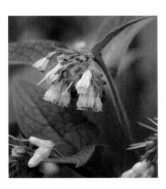

Comfrey

Botanical Name: *Symphytum* spp.

Family: Boraginaceae

Common Name(s): Russian comfrey, prickly comfrey, Quaker comfrey, "knitbone"

Perennial growth

Parts used: leaves and root

Uses: astringent, expectorant, healing broken bones, healing wounds, soothes skin, anti-inflammatory, stops bleeding

Harvest: Harvest young leaves in the spring for the most medicinal value, or harvest leaves as needed for general medicinal purposes.

History: Comfrey has had incredible medicinal uses for humans and livestock for centuries, though there is some controversy around it. It has been used since around 400 BC with a long history of benefits.

Greeks used comfrey much like we do today—to heal bones, wounds, and to stop heavy bleeding. Romans used comfrey to heal bones as well, and drank teas for stomach illness and bleeding. Comfrey is often called "knitbone" because it has been historically used to speed up the healing process of broken bones. Comfrey has been used as fodder for livestock and general livestock health. But the questioning of comfrey began in 1978 when a study found that rats that were fed comfrey developed liver tumors. Comfrey can absolutely be potentially toxic if not used properly. Today, we use comfrey cautiously but still know that it holds great medicinal benefits. Comfrey is most widely used to help speed up the healing process of broken bones. We also use comfrey externally on bruises, sores, and wounds.

How We Use It: We use comfrey mainly for its ability to stop bleeding and to speed up the healing process of broken bones. I create an infused oil or salve out of comfrey to keep on hand for these situations. Comfrey is also a fabulous herb to utilize in your garden. Create a tea with comfrey to fertilize your plants and encourage their growth. This works well for leafy green plants and herbs. You can also turn your comfrey tea concentrate into a spray.

Safety and Dosage: Comfrey shouldn't be used internally without supervision from a professional. Do not apply it to completely broken skin. Do not use when nursing. Use externally.

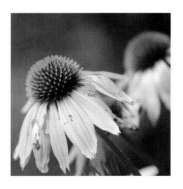

Echinacea

Botanical Name: *Echinacea purpurea* or *Echinacea angustifolia*

Family: Asteraceae

Common Name(s): purple coneflower

Perennial growth

Parts used: root, leaves, flowers

Uses: treats upper respiratory infections, natural cold remedy, treats yeast and fungal overgrowth, blood purifier, natural antibiotic, antibacterial

Harvest: The root is the most sought-after part of this herb; however, it takes a good three years of maturity before the root can be harvested. While you wait for the root, you can harvest the leaves and flower tops once they are in their prime.

Early morning harvest is best. Once the root matures, pull up the plant and dry the root on a drying rack or use fresh in your tincture or glycerite.

History: Echinacea is the very first herb I ever began growing here on my homestead. The Native Americans used echinacea extensively, along with black-eyed Susans, which are part of the same herb family. This herb was heavily relied upon for most ailments. Echinacea was used as a natural antibiotic, blood purifier, wound healer, and for ailments like bee stings, poisonous snakebites, gangrene, and more. Today we know that echinacea may not have that broad a range of medicinal benefits, though there is still much research to be done, but I can absolutely, without a doubt, tell you that it does fight infections, colds, and fungal overgrowth. Unfortunately, the Native American echinacea, *E. angustifolia*, was the most widely used throughout history, but in 1970 most of the research was done on *E. purpurea* due to mixed up seeds. Today, you can find both species; just make sure they are true to name.

It's a common misconception that echinacea prevents illness. For this outcome, you'd need something like astragalus or elderberry. Echinacea stimulates the immune system and helps support it, but it doesn't necessarily help prevent illness. Its job is to boost the immune system during illness or infection. At the very first sign of illness and infection, echinacea will lessen the symptoms and a full recovery will be much quicker than if you had waited until your symptoms were full blown. Echinacea also works well for yeast and ear infections.

How We Use It: Echinacea is one of the first tinctures you'll find on my medicine cabinet shelf. We use it at the first sign of cold symptoms. An oil can be made out of echinacea to rub around the ear for ear infections. We create mashes of leaves to put on wounds. I enjoy giving echinacea to my livestock as well. My meat rabbits especially enjoy echinacea leaves and flower tops as treats and monthly immunity boosters. Because rabbits are a prey animal, and they can be quite fragile, echinacea is high on the list of things I give them. Not only does it help boost immunity if something is incubating inside them, it also helps with any fungal or bacterial infections they may have going on that I haven't detected yet. Echinacea is great for the female farm dog that is prone to UTIs. We use it often for this very reason.

Safety and Dosage: Echinacea is typically made into a 1:5 tincture—5 mL (or 1 glass dropperful) of liquid can be taken 3–5 times a day until symptoms subside. Echinacea can be taken in a tea, 2–3 teaspoons of dried leaf/root. Avoid if you have a ragweed allergy. Avoid if you have an autoimmune disorder. Do not take for longer than eight consecutive weeks.

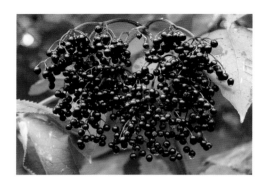

Elderberry

Botanical Name: *Sambucus nigra*

Family: Caprifoliaceae

Common Name(s): black elder, black elderberry, European elder

Perennial growth

Parts used: berries, flowers

Uses: supports immune health, treats flu and common cold, stimulant, relieves digestive issues, induces perspiration, antiviral

Harvest: Harvest flowers as soon as they open in the early summer. Harvest berries as soon as they turn a deep, dark purple, almost black.

History: People have used elderberry for the same thing throughout history: to boost the immune system and rid our bodies of the common cold and flu.

The leaves, stems, and roots of the elderberry plant can be poisonous and should be handled with care. This is why we use just the flowers and berries of the plant and cook them down to rid them of any poisonous components. Elderberries and flowers are most often used in tinctures and syrups as a preventative or as a healing agent for flu and colds.

How We Use It: Elderberry syrup was the very first medicinal herbal syrup that I ever made. I doubted it greatly, but when it worked on my then toddler, I sang its praises.

We use elderberry in tinctures, syrups, and even in our livestock herbal products. It boosts immunity and truly does lessen the symptoms of common cold and flu.

Safety and Dosage: Elderberry is generally considered safe; however, for those who have autoimmune disorders, speak with your doctor before using it, as immune stimulants can cause adverse reactions for you. Do not eat raw elderberries. Do not eat any of the elderberry plant. Syrup dosage: 1–3 tablespoons per day, three times a day, until symptoms subside. Or 2–3 teaspoons per day as a preventative. Tincture dosage: 30 drops three times a day until symptoms subside.

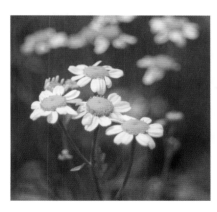

Feverfew

Botanical Name: *Chrysanthemum parthenium*

Family: Asteraceae

Common Name(s): feverfew, febrifuge plant

Biennial growth

Parts used: leaves, flowers

Uses: laxative, reduces fever, increases menstrual flow, pain reducer (specifically migraines and arthritis), anti-inflammatory

Harvest: You'll find feverfew growing in fields and even in the middle of old walkways if allowed to grow. Harvest the leaves and flowers once they mature. Dry and store in a cool, dry place.

History: Feverfew is most known for its fever-reducing properties, hence the name "feverfew." However, it's also known as a natural pain reliever, especially for migraines. The medicinal properties in feverfew react with the muscles of the body, causing them to relax, which in turn helps ease pain and migraines, especially migraines specific to stress and muscle spasms. Ancient Greeks used feverfew during childbirth to help with the delivery of afterbirth, as it caused the uterus to contract regularly. In the seventeenth century, it was claimed to heal toothaches. It was also said to help against vertigo, colic, kidney stones, and insect bites. In modern science, however, we still mainly use the herb as a natural pain reliever and fever reducer, or for conditions such as asthma, dizziness, dermatitis, or migraines.

How We Use It: I enjoy making a tincture out of feverfew flowers and leaves for migraines, respiratory issues, and fever.

Safety and Dosage: Women who are pregnant or nursing should not take feverfew. People who are allergic to ragweed and other plants in the ragweed family may have an allergic reaction to feverfew. A 1:5 tincture can be created with feverfew. Take 30 drops every 3–6 hours each day as needed. After taking for a week, slowly begin to discontinue use. Do not stop using abruptly, as this could cause headaches. Do not take aspirin or pain relievers while taking feverfew.

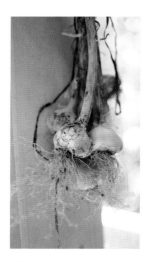

Garlic

Botanical Name: *Allium sativum*

Family: Liliaceae

Common Name(s): common garlic

Perennial growth

Parts used: Bulbs, scapes (culinary)

Uses: diuretic, expectorant, fever reducer, antispasmodic, stimulates digestive tract, regulates liver and gallbladder, reduces high cholesterol and blood pressure, boosts immune system, fights and treats infections

Harvest: Plant garlic bulbs in the fall for a spring harvest. When scapes turn yellow and begin to fall over, harvest garlic bulbs. Put on a drying rack and allow the bulbs to dry completely before storing. You can store the bulbs by braiding them and hanging them in the pantry or cellar, or you can turn the herb into homemade garlic powder by dehydrating them. The scapes can be harvested and eaten as a culinary delight, much like onion scapes.

History: Garlic has been cultivated so long that there's really no way to trace where it first began being used. Garlic has been used for its medicinal properties for centuries, and is still one of the most commonly known herbs for medicine and culinary uses today. In World War I, army doctors would use garlic to wash open wounds so that they wouldn't become infected. Garlic helps lower blood pressure and high cholesterol, and helps regulate blood circulation. It plays a powerful role in preventing multiple types of cancer. Through many scientific trials, garlic has been proven to be a powerful supplement when consumed through culinary medicine. Add garlic to your diet to help boost immunity, and increase your consumption of the herb during the winter months when you're more likely to need the immunity boost. Garlic has been used to help aid in digestive infections such as dysentery, typhoid, enteritis, and cholera.

How We Use It: Garlic is another herb that we add to our livestock's diet, as it is a powerful preventative. It also helps aid in the eradication of certain intestinal parasites, such as pinworms. Add garlic to your feed and waterers in bulb or powder form to boost immunity and ease digestion. Garlic is one of my favorite culinary herbs. I use it often in Italian dishes, soups, and stews, and when I make pickles and dilly beans. In the winter months, boosting our garlic intake through powdered capsules or simply by adjusting our diets helps us maintain healthy immune systems.

Safety and Dosage: For coughs, take grated garlic in honey or make a garlic syrup. Standard dose of garlic is up to 4 grams of fresh garlic each day. Take 20 drops of a 1:5 tincture three times a day as needed. Because garlic has a blood-thinning effect, avoid it if you are on blood thinners or have any condition that might be aggravated by this property. Otherwise, there are no known precautions with the culinary delivery of garlic.

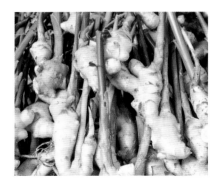

Ginger

Botanical Name: *Zingiber officinale*

Family: Zingiberaceae

Common Name(s): common ginger, shunthi

Perennial growth

Parts used: roots

Uses: appetite stimulant, reduces nausea and vomiting, stimulates veins and arteries, stimulates the heart, induces perspiration, relieves flatulence, soothes digestive tract, promotes circulation, soothes sore throat

Harvest: Harvest mature roots and use fresh or dried. Try not to harvest your original root planting, as it will offer new ginger for years to come. Much like turmeric, ginger can be grown in many climates, but it does present a challenge in colder climates. Start your ginger root plantings indoors in the winter months. Once the spring warmth is "here to stay," transplant your ginger to your garden. Ginger is a lot more forgiving than turmeric, and can be winterized in many climates after its first year of growth. Add deep mulch or straw after the first frost. If you fear it will be too cold, dig up the ginger after the first frost and store inside for the following year's root plantings.

History: Ginger is one of those herbs the Chinese have used throughout the centuries—like ginseng. Around 2000 BC, Emperor Shen Nong (the "Divine Farmer") wrote the Chinese herbal guide *Shen Nong Ben Cao King*, where ginger made its first appearance as an herb. We later see the herb used extensively throughout India and the Roman Empire. The Spanish were cultivating ginger in the sixteenth century, and ginger was introduced to the Americas, via Jamaica, in the sixteenth century as well. It rose to popularity quickly, mainly for its use in culinary dishes and baked goods but also for its ease of use as a medicinal herb.

Ginger is an herb that can be utilized well in food to help the body medicinally, while maintaining a delicious taste and aroma. Today, we use ginger most commonly to flavor drinks and dishes. But ginger can also be used for nausea and the digestive tract. Ginger is hot to the tongue, but has a citrus taste. It's best to use it in products rather than taking raw.

How We Use It: You'll find ginger in a lot of our tummy-soothing teas or herbal confectionaries. Ginger is a fabulous herb for morning sickness, stomach bugs, and to boost overall health. Homemade ginger ale is a hit, as are ginger chews!

Safety and Dosage: There are no known precautions to take with ginger, and it is generally considered safe to use. Use 2–3 drops of ginger essential oil topically or in a capsule or on a sugar cube; 2–3 teaspoon (or more) of dried ginger can be used in a tea with 8 ounces of hot water. Ginger tinctures can be taken as needed, with the general rule of 30 drops three times a day.

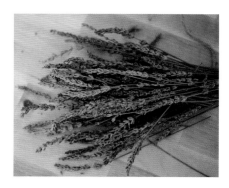

Lavender

Botanical Name: *Lavendula augustifolia*

Family: Lamiaceae

Common Name(s): common lavender, English Lavender, true lavender

Perennial growth

Parts used: flowers, sometimes leaves

Uses: antispasmodic, sedative, digestive aid, calming, soothing for burns and bug bites, disinfectant, antibacterial

Harvest: Harvest lavender in the early morning before the dew evaporates from the flowers. This ensures that the volatile oils still remain intact within the plant. Harvest lavender flowers before they open, cutting the stem at the next set of leaves closest to the bottom of the plant. Pull lavender flowers off of stems and store in an airtight container. Keeping the lavender flowers on the stem and hanging to dry also works, but it does begin to lose its scent and medicinal properties much more rapidly.

History: Lavender is a Mediterranean herb that derives from the Latin word meaning "to wash." Lavender was often hung in bathhouses and other areas for its aromatic properties. In the Middle Ages, lavender was thought to be an herb of love since it was considered an aphrodisiac. Lavender was even used as a disinfectant for wounds. Lavender produces an oil that can treat insomnia, enhance mood and calmness, aid in intestinal problems, and is antibacterial and antiseptic. Lavender is great for healing the skin, soothing bug bites and wounds. It's also a great aid in digestion when taken as an herbal tea. Culinarily, lavender is most notably used in the Westernized Herbes de Provence spice blend, which originated in Europe. Lavender can also be used in many baked goodies, like shortbread cookies and lemon pound cake.

How We Use It: Lavender is one of those herbs that I grow because it's beautiful. The scent of lavender essential oil is way too much for me, but the scent of fresh lavender flowers is one of the most decadent scents I've ever smelled. I use large lavender bundles throughout the barn and chicken coop to freshen up the space and set a mood of calmness for the animals. I also enjoy making lavender lotions and even add lavender into some of my salves for its healing properties and as a natural antibacterial cream. I enjoy lavender bouquets in my home. I'm also particularly fond of lavender-lemon pound cake (see recipe on page 229). I use lavender essential oil in blends and directly on bug bites and other wounds to help soothe and disinfect.

Safety and Dosage: Steep 1–2 teaspoons of dried lavender leaves in 8 ounces of boiling water to make an herbal tea infusion. Lavender is generally considered to be a safe herb, and there are no known reasons to avoid it.

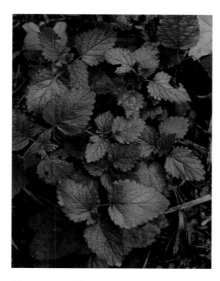

Lemon Balm

Botanical Name: *Melissa officinalis*

Family: Lamiaceae

Common Name(s): balm, lemon balm, Melissa balm

Perennial growth

Parts used: leaves

Uses: aids in digestion, antioxidant, calms nervous system, aids in depression, antiviral, antibacterial, enhances memory, stimulates the thyroid, promotes fertility

Harvest: Harvest lemon balm in the early morning so that the oils are not dried up on the leaves. Use fresh, or dry within two days and store in an airtight container. Lemon balm will spread rapidly if allowed to go to seed, ensuring lemon balm for all eternity!

History: Lemon balm is one of the first herbs notably used by botanist and Greek physician Dioscorides, who wrote the herbal *De Materia Medica.* The ancient Greeks and Romans, and people throughout the Middle Ages, used lemon balm for insect bites and stings, to aid in digestion, to balance mood, and to promote sleep. Lemon balm stimulates the thyroid, eases digestion and digestive irritabilities, calms the nervous system, works as a sedative, promotes a sense of calm and balance, relieves stress, and is generally used for overall health. Lemon balm has been said to help with fertility. Lemon balm is also used as an insect deterrent, deterring mosquitoes and other unwanted pests when planted around outbuildings and in the garden.

How We Use It: Lemon balm is one of my favorite herbs. It's exceptionally easy to grow, and it spreads like wildfire when allowed to go to seed, much like peppermint and spearmint. I plant lemon balm around my garden, around the garden pond, under the hammock, and around outbuildings to deter pests and insects, especially mosquitoes. It has a lemony flavor that works fabulously in drinks and even for cleaning since it has antibacterial properties. Lemon balm essential oil is one of those miracle oils that can heal viral and bacterial issues in the body, so we keep this on hand for those moments when we need to hit an ailment quickly and effectively.

Safety and Dosage: Steep 2–4 grams of fresh or dried lemon balm in 8 ounces of boiling water to make an herbal tea infusion. Use 2–3 drops lemon balm essential oil at a time, externally. A little goes a long way. Do not use if pregnant or nursing.

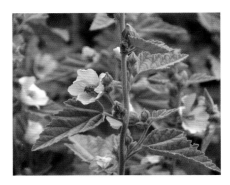

Marshmallow

Botanical Name: *Althaea officinalis*

Family: Malvaceae

Common Name(s): althaea, althea, marshmallow plant

Perennial growth

Parts used: leaves, roots, flowers

Uses: anti-inflammatory, diuretic, expectorant, soothes skin, urinary tract anti-inflammatory, heals wounds, respiratory aid, reduces coughing

Harvest: The mucilage content in the root is best when harvested in the fall and winter. Harvest the leaves and flowers as they mature.

History: Marshmallow root is probably one of the most popular staple herbs throughout the history of herbalism, dating all the way back to the ninth century BC. The Greek physician Hippocrates valued it as a wound treatment. Dioscorides valued it in a vinegar infusion to help with toothaches and soothe insect stings. Herbalists throughout generations have valued this herb for its ability to soothe sore throats and coughs, and to heal urinary tract irritation and inflammation. Perhaps today the most popular use of marshmallow is to help reduce coughing and inflammation in the respiratory tract. It is a common ingredient in cough syrups.

How We Use It: Marshmallow . . . no, not the kind you put on top of your hot chocolate. We like marshmallow because it helps soothe sore throats and respiratory inflammation, and that's really what it does best! This is our "wintertime" herb to keep on hand. We especially love it in a marshmallow-infused hot chocolate (see recipe on page 230). Marshmallow is sometimes best made into a poultice and rubbed on the area that needs healing or support, but works wonders when ingested as well. When creating a poultice, you'll notice that the marshmallow becomes gel-like. We use it internally and externally, often at the same time for the same issue.

Safety and Dosage: There are no known precautions with this herb, and it is generally considered safe to consume. Tincture dosage: 30 drops three times a day. Syrup dosage: 10 mL three times a day. Steep 1–2 teaspoons of dried marshmallow in a tea or drink.

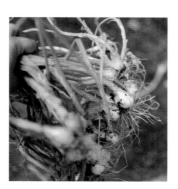

Onion

Botanical Name: *Allium cepa*

Family: Liliaceae

Common Name(s): standard onion

Perennial growth (or biennial if allowed to go to seed or replanted)

Parts used: bulbs and scapes

Uses: antibacterial, antifungal, antiseptic, diuretic, expectorant, antispasmodic

Harvest: There are many different ways to harvest onions, depending on what you're using them for. To harvest mature bulbs, wait until your onion tops have fallen over and are yellowed. Leave your onions out in a safe, dry place. Once dry, you can braid your onions and store them in a root cellar or hang them in a dark area of your home. To harvest scapes, simply cut as you wish, much like chives. Keep in mind, however, that this may cause harm to your onion bulb.

History: Onions were widely used as a medicinal herb from the beginning of time, dating as far back as the Egyptians in 3200 BC. In more recent history, they were used to clean and sterilize the wounds of soldiers in the Civil War, since they have antiseptic properties. For people who tend to eat high-fat diets, onions can actually help lower cholesterol and clean out arteries or fatty deposits. Experiments have even shown that onion extract can lower high blood pressure. Onions can be used to prevent infection in open wounds. A syrup made from onions can act as a natural cough syrup, though it goes down better when mixed with honey. Many people also believe that placing a slice of onion on your feet at night while you sleep can help pull sickness out of your body, especially the common cold. While it hasn't been scientifically proven, I personally know many who claim this to be true. Onions are most widely used as a culinary herb in many dishes.

How We Use It: My main use for onions is in culinary dishes, stocks, and broth. Onions are one of those herbs that I can grow, harvest, dry, and store, long term, so that whenever I want to use them medicinally, I can simply pull a bulb from my pantry. I enjoy using onions in just about anything I cook, if we're being honest— from chicken pot pie and meat stocks, to squash casserole and tomato pie. Onions are just good eatin'!

Safety and Dosage: There are no known issues with onion; however, anything in large quantities can cause an upset stomach.

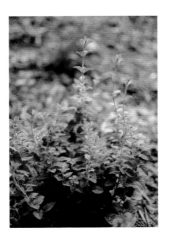

Oregano

Botanical Name: *Origanum vulgare*

Family: Lamiaceae

Common Name(s): wild marjoram

Perennial growth

Parts used: Leaves and flowering stems

Uses: antibacterial, aching muscles, bug bites, detoxifying, toothache, respiratory, antibiotic, expectorant, regulates menstrual cycle, reduces colic

Harvest: Sprigs of the plant can be harvested throughout the spring, summer, and fall. Simply clip larger sprigs down to just above the final set of new leaves. You'll have an endless amount of oregano throughout the season.

History: Oregano has quite an interesting history that dates back to the Roman Empire and beyond. The name "oregano" means "joy of the mountains" and was often used in wedding ceremonies to adorn the head of the bride. The Greeks made poultices with oregano and placed them on aching muscles, wounds, and bites. Since oregano is naturally antibacterial, it has been used to treat illnesses and infections for centuries. Most often, the oil is used to treat whatever the issue may be as a more aggressive approach. There are different types of oregano, but *Origanum vulgare* is the most popular and widely used for medicinal and culinary purposes. This is the oregano that I stick with for all of my needs. If you're looking for a boost in culinary flavor, try *O. heracleoticum (O. hirtum)* or *Lippia graveolens*, also known as Mexican oregano or Puerto Rican oregano, respectively.

How We Use It: Around our homestead, we use oregano in our livestock feed and water to help prevent bacterial infections and outbreaks of disease. The oil can be used on cuts and wounds to deter bacterial infection. Place a drop of the oil on an abscessed or aching tooth to help relieve the pain. We also use it to make an awesome pizza sauce and other Italian dishes! Using oregano culinarily is actually the best way to consume it. It increases the detoxification process of the body and is great as an herbal preventative.

Safety and Dosage: Oregano is a tonic herb, which means you can typically consume as much of it as you'd like when used culinarily. With essential oils, we only use 2–3 drops per use. Steep 2–3 teaspoons of dried oregano in a cup of hot water to make a tea infusion. There are no known safety precautions with oregano when consumed culinarily, which should be your main way of consuming it.

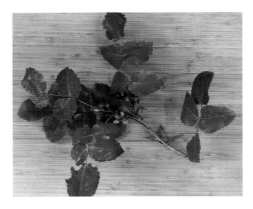

Oregon Grape Root

Botanical Name: *Mahonia aquifolium*

Family: Berberidaceae

Common Name(s): Oregon grape, holly-leaved barberry, mountain grape, Oregon barberry, Oregon grapeholly

Perennial growth

Parts used: roots

Uses: antibacterial, antibiotic, eczema, ear infections, parasites, sinus infections, acne, diarrhea, promotes good liver function, stimulates bile secretion, purifies the spleen and blood, psoriasis

Harvest: Oregon grape root grows mostly in the wild, though it can be cultivated in the homesteader's garden where it doesn't grow natively. Harvest the root of mature plants in the late fall or winter, after the berries have developed. You can grab the berries and plant them where you've harvested, much like we do ginseng, so that a new plant grows the following year.

History: Oregon grape root is a fairly new herb on the scene in North America, although it isn't new at all. It works much the way goldenrod does; therefore we see it beginning to soar in popularity. Historically, Oregon grape root was used by Native Americans for food and medicine. The berries were used to make jelly and wine. The root was used as medicine to cure ulcers, arthritis, skin conditions, and kidney issues. Frontiersmen learned of Oregon grape root from Native Americans, and in the 1800s, it rose quickly in popularity to treat skin conditions, jaundice, and hemorrhaging. In modern medicine, this herb is used primarily for skin conditions, especially psoriasis and eczema. But while it is medicinally beneficial, it should never be used as a preventative, as it can be toxic. It should only be used internally when an illness occurs or for topical treatment.

How We Use It: This herb is extremely new to the Fewell homestead, and I'll admit, it isn't something we use often. However, it's one of those herbs I like to keep around for friends and family that deal with skin irritations, and for our livestock as well. It is a powerfully aggressive antibacterial and antiparasitic for humans and animals alike.

Safety and Dosage: Oregon grape root should not be used as a preventative as it can be toxic. Long-term use can cause vitamin B deficiency. Avoid if you are pregnant, breastfeeding, have diabetes, or have a history of stroke, hypertension, or glaucoma. Tincture dosage: 30 drops three times a day (again, only when ailing).

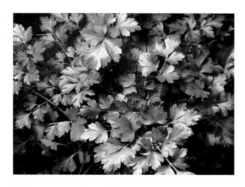

Parsley

Botanical Name: *Petroselinum crispum*

Family: Apiaceae

Common Name(s): parsley

Annual growth (biennial growth after it goes to seed in second year)

Parts used: leaves, roots, seeds

Uses: mostly culinary, increases menstrual flow, high in vitamins A, B, and C, high in calcium and iron

Harvest: Harvest parsley as needed. In its second year, parsley will often bolt and go to seed.

History: In ancient Greece, parsley was used for funeral ceremonies, wreaths, and garlands. It was often given to livestock to help increase stamina. It was used to help cleanse the kidneys and liver, but in modern medicine, it doesn't demonstrate much medicinal benefit. Today, we use parsley in culinary dishes more than anything else.

How We Use It: I enjoy using parsley as a companion plant in the garden since it specifically attracts swallowtail butterflies and enhances the fragrance of some cut flowers. We give parsley to our livestock as a highly effective boost in vitamins and minerals.

Safety and Dosage: Because parsley isn't necessarily a medicinal herb, it can be consumed as needed. Do avoid giving it to livestock in extra large quantities, as it could lower blood pressure too much when consumed in a medicinal amount.

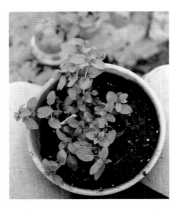

Peppermint

Botanical Name: *Mentha piperita*

Family: Lamiaceae

Common Name(s): peppermint

Perennial growth

Parts used: leaves

Uses: antiseptic, antispasmodic, aids in digestion, natural pain killer (externally), fever reducer, reduces nervousness, reduces headache, promotes clear breathing

Harvest: Clip sprigs all season long by cutting the largest sprigs first, down to the ground. You can use fresh or dehydrate for longer storage. Allow to go to seed for exponential growth each year; however, it can be invasive if not strategically placed or cut back each year.

History: Peppermint is probably one of the most recognizable herbs based on its scent. Most people who've never had any training in herbs can spot it by simply rubbing its leaves and inhaling. Peppermint played a large role in ancient Egypt, Rome, and Grecian cultures. It was, and still is, most widely used to aid in digestion and tummy troubles. Drinking peppermint in a tea or drink (or taking it in capsules) helps with nausea, indigestion, heartburn, and upset stomach. Applying peppermint or peppermint essential oil (diluted) to the skin can help with inflammation and sunburn. When inhaled, peppermint clears breathing during colds, asthmatic conditions, and respiratory infections. The essential oil is most commonly used for headaches and to reduce fever or to create a cooling effect during a hot summer day.

How We Use It: I keep peppermint on hand at all times, in dried and essential oil form. We use peppermint essential oil to reduce fever, cool us on hot days, and reduce headaches, and I even use it in peppermint treats during the holidays. Peppermint essential oil also makes an incredible toothpaste or tooth powder. We go through several bottles of peppermint essential oil each year for this very reason. Brewing peppermint in a tea is essential in our household when we've eaten something that didn't agree with us, or when we've simply overeaten. It helps us with digestive issues and is a natural anti-inflammatory for the bowels. During times where my gluten sensitivity flares up, peppermint tea is necessary for my comfort. I also enjoy using peppermint in tinctures and iced tea.

Safety and Dosage: Peppermint is not an herb to be used every single day. When using it to treat an ailment or issue, use for 8–12 days, then stop for one week before resuming. Steep 2–3 teaspoons of dried leaves to make a cup of tea. Take 3–4 drops of essential oil in a capsule to relieve digestive issues. For a 1:5 tincture ratio, 10 mL can be taken up to three times each day during use. If you have gallstones, consult a professional first before using. Otherwise, there are no safety precautions with peppermint.

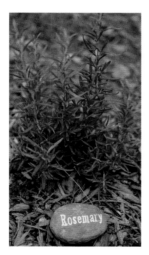

Rosemary

Botanical Name: *Rosmarinus officinalis*

Family: Lamiaceae

Common Name(s): standard rosemary, common rosemary

Perennial growth

Parts used: leaves, flowering tops

Uses: enhances brain function, boosts memory, reduces headaches, reduces stress, antispasmodic, promotes liver function, aids in digestion and bile creation, raises blood pressure and improves circulation, external use for arthritis and eczema

Harvest: Harvest entire springs of rosemary as needed, cutting down almost to the ground when harvesting.

History: Rosemary is one of the most widely popular herbs throughout the centuries. In the Middle Ages, men and women would place rosemary under their pillows to ward off evil spirits and illness. At one point in history, most brides would wear rosemary dipped in scented water, either as head or neck wreaths or in their bouquets. And oftentimes, rosemary was known as the remembrance or friendship herb. Today, we use rosemary mainly as a culinary herb, but it does have some medicinal purpose as well. It has been recommended in the treatment of depression, headaches, stress, arthritis, and digestion. Be careful with the amount you ingest, however, as it can be toxic in extremely high doses.

How We Use It: If you need to grow an herb that won't die on you immediately—grow rosemary, although, it can be a bit harder to grow in colder climates. Rosemary is one of my favorite herbs to cook with, and it is fragrant in the beautiful aromatic essential oil that we love so much. Sometimes I add rosemary to my livestock feed to aid in digestion, liver function, and during stressful times. It's also a great herb to ease tension and headaches.

Safety and Dosage: Add 1–2 teaspoons dried rosemary to 1 cup boiling water for infused tea. Tincture dosage: 20 drops of rosemary tincture up to twice a day. Use rosemary essential oil sparingly, or up to 2 drops.

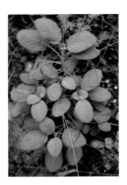

Sage

Botanical Name: *Salvia officinalis*

Family: Lamiaceae

Common Name(s): common sage, garden sage, Dalmatian sage

Perennial growth

Parts used: leaves and stems

Uses: antispasmodic, astringent, reduction of perspiration, treats menopausal women, aids in digestion, helps treat viral and fungal infections

Harvest: Harvest the velvety leaves as needed, or cut full stems off right above the last small set of new leaves.

History: Sage was used extensively throughout history, especially by Arabians and throughout the Middle Ages, for warts, seizures, measles, and worms. Native Americans mixed sage with bear grease to create a salve to treat skin irritations and sores. Sage has also been used to dry up the flow of mother's milk, and to stop excessive urination, saliva, and perspiration. Sage is most often used in meals all across the world, especially for sausage mixtures. Today, we continue to use sage extensively in culinary dishes. We also use it to help menopausal women with night sweats and hot flashes. And it treats viral and fungal infections. You can find sage in cleaning products and modern cosmetics as well.

How We Use It: Sage is really a homestead staple, especially if you cook. Sage is one of the main herbs in sausage, and we all know homesteaders love sausage! Sage is such a beautiful aromatic herb that I love to have some sitting on my counter for quick use or just for the scent. We cook with it often, and I use it in my livestock feed, for dairy animals going dry, and for those "time of the month" night sweats. It also works well in deodorants and salves.

Safety and Dosage: Avoid if pregnant or breastfeeding except for culinary use. Add 2–3 teaspoons dried sage per 8 ounces of boiling water to make a tea infusion. Do not take medicinal amounts of sage for an extended period of time as it could cause toxicity.

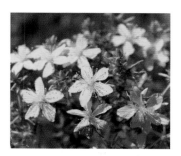

St. John's Wort

Botanical Name: *Hypericum perforatum*

Family: Clusiaceae

Common Name(s): St. John's wort

Perennial growth

Parts used: flowers and leaves

Uses: antidepressant, antibacterial, astringent, soothe the digestive tract, sedative, pain reliever, anti-inflammatory

Harvest: Leaves and flowers should be harvested at peak season, typically in July and August.

History: This herb is another example of old folk medicine, where users of the herb believed it had the power to ward off evil spirits. For over two thousand years, herbalists have used St. John's wort to help with digestive upset, pain relief, and to enhance mood and emotions.

How We Use It: Today, we use it for many of the same reasons and much more extensively for general health and well-being. In fact, it is one of the most-studied herbs when it comes to emotional support and is often used as an antidepressant. This herb can also be used by women suffering from menopausal symptoms, women suffering from their monthly cycle, people who deal with skin irritations like psoriasis, and even those who have nerve pain and irritable bowel syndrome.

Safety and Dosage: While this herb seems like a miracle herb, it does come with side effects that should be noted. We use this herb mostly in a tea (minimal dosage) or for skin irritations. When taken in proper dosages, please understand that this herb is absolutely safe and easy to use, but there are precautions to take while using it. Do not use during phototherapy, and if you are a fair-skinned person, avoid excessive exposure to sunlight while using this herb. St. John's wort can interact with other medications, so please consult a professional before using. Suggested dosages are 300–900 mL by mouth twice a day for two weeks. Can be taken for up to twelve weeks, but consult with a professional for extended use. Tincture dosage: a 1:5 ratio, 30 drops per day.

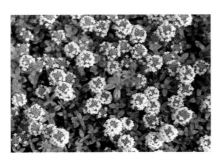

Thyme

Botanical Name: *Thymus vulgaris*

Family: Lamiaceae

Common Name(s): garden thyme, common thyme

Perennial growth

Parts used: leaves

Uses: vermifuge (parasites), antibacterial, antiseptic, antispasmodic, relieves cough, expectorant, regulates gut flora, relieves upper respiratory infection, increases DHA (omega-3 fatty acid) in the brain and heart

Harvest: Cut sprigs of thyme throughout the season, cutting larger sprigs down to the ground first. Harvest in batches by only cutting stems halfway, in order to allow the thyme to grow all season long.

History: Thyme has an extensive history in culinary and medicinal uses. It's one of those herbs you *have* to grow on your homestead, because there are *so many* good and amazing things about it. In the medieval era, knights would wear sprigs of thyme on their armor, given to them by women of nobility, as a sign of courage and bravery. It's also believed that the scent of thyme would give them strength during a battle. The Greeks used thyme for nervous conditions, the Egyptians used it in their embalming rituals, and it was used in medieval Europe because it was thought to ward off plagues. Thyme has scientifically been known to help with respiratory infections, especially whooping cough and respiratory syncytial virus. In fact, often the taste in cough syrups comes from the thyme used in the syrup. Thyme naturally rids the body of parasites in the digestive tract and regulates the gut flora.

How We Use It: During the winter months when coughs and colds are most prevalent, I create a tea with thyme to help aid with coughs and respiratory ailments. Thyme essential oil can be used for the tummy and digestive issues when used externally on the feet or rubbed on the belly. And thyme is well suited for culinary medicine. I also add thyme to our livestock feed as a natural preventative. It also naturally rids livestock of internal parasites, especially hookworms.

Safety and Dosage: Thyme tea should contain 1–2 teaspoons of dried leaves per 8 ounces of water. Thyme essential oil can be used externally (2–3 drops) or internally (1–2 drops). Women who are pregnant should use the essential oil with caution.

For a 1:5 tincture, take 20–30 drops three times a day as needed. Individuals with a history of thyroid disease should not consume thyme in large quantities.

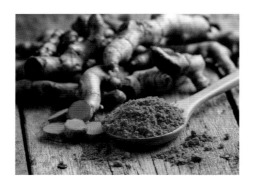

Turmeric

Botanical Name: *Curcuma longa*

Family: Zingiberaceae

Common Name(s): common turmeric, Indian saffron, yellow ginger

Perennial growth

Parts used: roots

Uses: anti-inflammatory, joint health, antioxidant, blood purifier, blood thinner, arthritis

Harvest: Harvest the root of turmeric when fully mature. Leave some root behind for perennial growth. Use fresh turmeric in culinary dishes or fire cider, or dry turmeric and grind into a powder for future use. While turmeric is easy to grow in most seasonal climates, it is a bit difficult in climates that are cold during most growing seasons. Turmeric has been grown as far north as New England, with deep mulch winterizing in the winter months. You can also dig up the root and bring it indoors to use or store, then replant it in the spring. You'll need to start turmeric indoors or in a greenhouse in the spring months. Once the weather remains fairly warm, you can plant it in your garden. It will expand and grow quickly. Dig the turmeric root back up or try winterizing it with mulch and straw after the first frost.

History: Turmeric has been used throughout the ages, mainly in Indian culinary dishes and as an anti-inflammatory. Curcumin is the antioxidant compound that is found in turmeric that helps make the herb beneficial to the body. It is widely used for its ability to promote joint mobility and decrease inflammation. This is why it makes it such a great herb to use, especially if you have rheumatoid arthritis. This herb also pairs really well with Mexican and Indian dishes, and is a great herb to use in livestock feed.

How We Use It: I feel like turmeric is constantly being used in our home. I sprinkle some on the dog food, livestock feed, and in our own dishes. Turmeric can easily be used in almost any dish. It's truly a culinary herb that can double as a medicinal one with little effort. We especially take turmeric capsules during times of joint inflammation or when we've worked hard and have pain throughout the body.

Safety and Dosage: There are no known precautions with this herb, and it is generally safe to use.

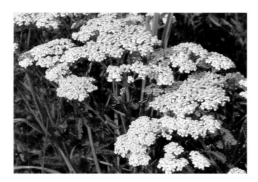

Yarrow

Botanical Name: *Achillea millefolium*

Family: Asteraceae

Common Name(s): standard yarrow, milfoil

Perennial growth

Parts used: leaves, flowers, and stems

Uses: anti-inflammatory, stops bleeding, heals wounds, soothes skin, anti-anxiety, antibacterial, antispasmodic, lowers blood pressure, aids in cardiovascular health

Harvest: Harvest leaves, flower heads, and stems when the flower is in full bloom.

History: Yarrow has been used as a medicinal herb and as a dietary herb for centuries, dating all the way back to 1200 BC. Oftentimes, yarrow was used to make beer in place of hops. According to folk legend, the Greek warrior Achilles would use yarrow to treat his soldiers' wounds, hence the botanical name, *Achillea millefolium.*

How We Use It: Yarrow leaves and flower heads can be eaten and cooked much like spinach. It is a fabulous herb for asthmatic relief and general respiratory health. It is also used to heal wounds, help with anxiety, reduce muscle spasms, and to lower blood pressure.

Safety and Dosage: Yarrow can be made into a tea infusion, tincture, or used in a compress. A 1:5 tincture can be taken up to three times a day, 30 drops each dosage. Steep 1–3 teaspoons of dried yarrow in a cup of hot water. Do not use if you are pregnant or nursing unless told otherwise by a healthcare professional. Otherwise, this herb is considered safe for general consumption and there are no known precautions.

DON'T GET OVERWHELMED

While this list may seem massive, you'll likely find that you don't need all of the herbs that are listed. As I mentioned before, choosing the top five herbs that you'll need will be more than enough during your first year of herb gardening. As your herbal knowledge expands, so will the list of herbs that you grow. Just because I choose to have certain herbs in my pantry doesn't mean I use them all of the time, or that they are in my pantry every single day. This is why we choose to create things like tinctures and herbal honeys, so that we can harvest batches of herbs from our gardens and preserve them in products that will last more than a year.

Study this list of herbs and use it as a reference for years to come. And make sure you use this list when referencing the recipes and information throughout the rest of this book. Referring back to this list will help you create your own herbal products for your specific needs.

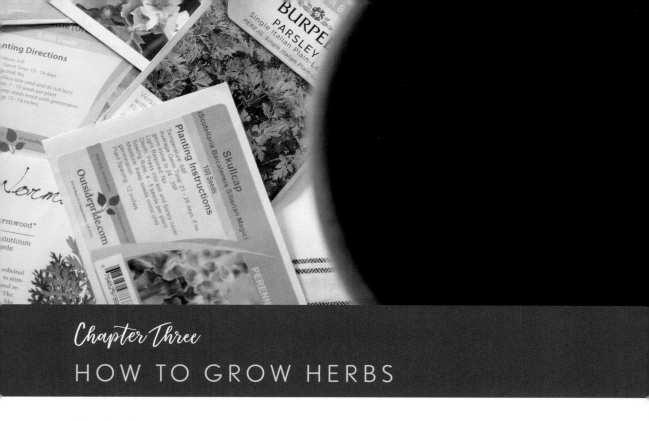

Chapter Three

HOW TO GROW HERBS

Most herbs are pretty forgiving, but there's a few things you'll need to think about before you begin digging into the dirt. Region, soil fertility, sunlight, and space limitations are things to take into consideration. Otherwise, you could just be wasting your time by throwing plants in the ground and praying they'll produce. Ask me how I know . . . never mind, just don't.

KNOW YOUR REGION AND ZONE

Every single region has a different zone number and climate. You'll need to consider this when choosing your herbs, just as you would your vegetables. Generally, if you're in a super cold climate, you want to make sure the plants you're planting in the ground are cold hardy (like garlic, thyme, and sage). If you're in a humid and hot climate, there are some herbs you'll need to keep out of direct sunlight in order to compensate for the heat (like cilantro and lemon balm). Or, you may just want to plant them in containers so that you can move your herbs with, or away from, the sunlight.

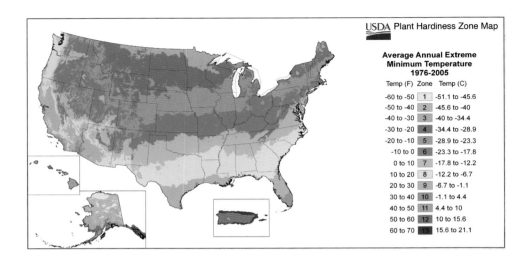

Every herb that you purchase, whether from seed or grown in a nursery, will come with instructions on the best time to plant that herb, and what the sunlight and watering routine should be. That little plastic thing that sticks up in the container that we all like to toss to the side while planting—it's actually useful! Who knew? Adjust those instructions according to your zone and climate.

KNOW YOUR SOIL

I could go into this long speech about how you should check the pH levels in your soil, but that would make me a hypocrite. I have never, in all the years I've been gardening, ever checked the pH levels in my soil. That's not to say that I won't ever do it, but I've yet to have a reason to do it. However, if you want to do so, then here's the lowdown.

What is soil pH? Soil pH is a measure of the acidity and alkalinity in your soil. The pH levels range from 0 to 14, with 7 being neutral, below 7 being acidic, and above 7 being alkaline. You typically want most soil to be between 5.5 and 7 pH. People who live in sandy or desert areas will have a bigger issue with evening out pH levels than those who do not. Some herbs, like mint, can even go as high as

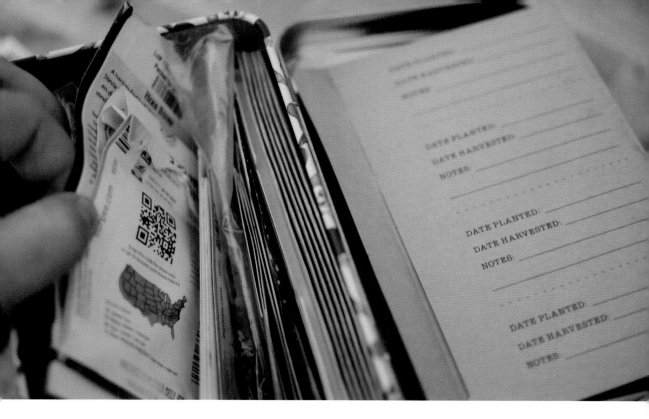

8. But honestly, each plant can adapt differently with proper soil fertility, which shouldn't be confused with pH levels.

You want to know what I do? I turn my soil over, and if it's dry, or not a deep, rich color, I throw some compost on it, cover it with leaf and organic matter, and let it sit the entire winter. Actually, let me just tell you how to get the richest soil you've ever had, and I promise, if you do it, you'll be able to grow just about anything. And most likely, you'll never have a reason to check your pH levels.

HOW TO "GET RICH" SOIL

This will all depend on the season you're in. Ideally, this "get rich" soil starts best in the late fall. The goal is to continuously add organic matter and material to your garden space. This allows you to create a rich soil with depth. It encourages good bacteria and earthworms to make their home there. And with a little tending, any

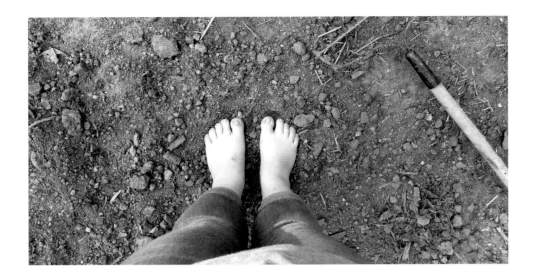

homesteader can have the richest soil ever. The key to it all is keeping your soil covered, not constantly exposing it to the harsh elements and sunlight.

Step 1: Kill the Grass

When you've decided where you want your garden space to be (in full sunlight), you'll need to make a mental or physical outline of it. If the area is a grassy area, or a lawn, then your first step is to lay down a dark-colored heavy duty tarp where you want your garden to be. Be sure to secure your tarp by placing heavy rocks on it so that the wind doesn't blow it around. Over a two- to three-week time period, leaving the tarp in the same place will kill all of the grass beneath the tarp and leave you with a brand new canvas to plant herbs in. This is a much more efficient option that trying to pull up all the grass with your tiller.

Step 2: Compost

Once your garden area is bare and ready to go, you can do one of two things. You can leave it bare and begin the composting process directly on top of the newly barren soil (this is a longer process), or you can till the area and begin your composting process immediately. You can learn more about these in-depth processes in the till and no-till method sections coming up next.

We choose to till our ground and begin the process immediately. This process can be started in the spring or the fall, whereas the first method mentioned (no tilling, just layering) takes an entire season before you can use it. We'll go over both methods. We actually use both methods, but always till first and layer compost onto our soil over the winter months.

Your goal is to continuously build up your soil. Your soil is never "always ready" to be planted in. This looks a lot like adding compost into your soil (like manure and homemade compost) in the spring when you are tilling the ground, and over-wintering your garden soil by placing a deep layer of organic matter (like leaves, pine needles, thick organic mulch) on top of it during the dormant months. Either way, adding a rich layer of compost or manure every so often really bulks up that soil. It is continuously building and shifting!

The Till Method. Till (either with a rototiller or hand tiller) the area that you've chosen for your new garden bed. Going over the space a few times and removing clumps of weeds, grass, or dirt will save you time in the long run. Make sure your soil is nice and "fluffy," because you'll be adding compost to it shortly. The fluffier and more fine the tilled soil, the easier it is to work with.

Once completely tilled, add a healthy layer of natural compost and manure. You can purchase bags of organic compost from your local farm or hardware store, or you can use your own fresh compost or manure.

Now that you're all tilled, composted, and manured (and maybe a little stinky!), next comes the one thing that will save your life as a gardener. **Mulch.** That's right, you're going to throw down a thick ol' layer of mulch, and that stuff is going to seal in all that rich dirt that you just labored over. Mulch helps your soil retain moisture, but it also helps generate and retain heat during those colder spring nights. If you do nothing else, don't forget the mulch.

A thin layer of mulch will do just fine for yearly maintenance after you've planted, but for the first year, a couple of inches is best. If you get organic mulch (which includes things like compost, leaves, and bark), this mulch will break down over the season and enrich your soil. If you get inorganic mulch, which is like regular landscaping mulch, it won't break down as quickly, but it does hold in a lot more moisture. We use both on our homestead—it just depends on what's on sale that week! Sometimes we use both at the same time by putting down a layer of organic mulch first, then inorganic mulch. Ultimately, you could use wood chips as well, but they take longer to break down and can invite more pests like termites and fire ants.

Best manure ever!

Straight rabbit manure is the best manure you'll ever find. The first year I used our homestead rabbit manure in our garden beds, our earthworms went from tiny little worms to the size of baby snakes in one year. I literally jumped back when I turned the soil over that spring because I thought snakes were coming after me! The difference in fertility was incredible.

The No-Till Method. The no-till method is very similar to the till method, except you don't till the ground and there's a little more layering. This is a pretty big movement in some gardening groups and is often referred to as the "Back to Eden" garden style. We've used it in the past, and it will work for many areas, but if you're a procrastinator like me, the till method works better.

The no-till method is best begun in the fall or winter. This allows the organic matter to break down before springtime planting. The goal is not to actually dig into the soil but to allow the organic matter to sit on top of the soil. This is beneficial for those who are disciplined enough to keep up with it, but for those of us who want a quicker and equally efficient method, the till method works just as well.

The no-till method is fabulous because you aren't disturbing the soil at all. Instead of tilling into the land, you're leaving the land alone and building the soil on top.

You'll begin by placing down your tarp or a layer of cardboard. This kills your grass as it does with the till method. After two weeks, you'll take the tarp up and begin building your soil. If you used cardboard, you can start building immediately right on top of the cardboard, as the cardboard will break down and serves as an excellent grass and weed barrier.

From this point, it's simple. You put down a healthy, thick layer of manure and compost, a layer of wood chips or a thick (6-plus-inch) layer of straw, and another layer of manure. This will begin to break down over the fall and winter months, leaving you with a healthy rich soil to dig right into that spring. Water your layered garden each week to help activate the manure to begin breaking down the wood chips and organic matter beneath it. You'll still need to add another layer of wood chips or mulch to your garden after you plant in the spring in order to retain moisture.

Implementing Both Methods. We use both methods in the fall and spring. In the spring we till our ground with the till method. In the fall, once everything has been harvested, we feed our soil with manure, compost, and a thick layer of mulch. This protects our soil from the harsh winter temperatures and continues to enrich the permaculture and good bacterial environment that we've created. This also helps us build another fertile layer of soil for the following year.

Either method is completely fine to do, but we believe that implementing both methods in different seasons is best. Both of these methods are essential to creating healthy, nutrient-dense herbs. While some herbs grow better in different soil types, every herb I've ever planted in this natural permaculture-type environment has thrived. If your garden environment and foundation is healthy and thriving with good microbes and bacteria, you can grow just about anything, within reason.

Step 3: Finalize with Fertilizer

This step is optional, but once I've planted my plants, I like to add a layer of blood meal around them to help fertilize and maintain good soil health. It's not pretty smelling but it sure does produce amazing plants.

DIFFERENT PLACES TO PLANT HERBS

Not everyone can, or wants to, grow herbs in their garden, though I highly recommend it. But maybe you have space limitations or simply want to try growing culinary herbs first. Or maybe it's a soil issue. Some people may need to grow in raised beds or containers. Baby steps are always wonderful, and small spaces can be utilized as well. Knowing your soil and your area is essential. The mere fact that you want to learn to grow and utilize herbs says a lot about how much and how quickly you'll take on the big garden. Either way, there are a lot of different ways and areas where you can plant herbs.

You can grow herbs just about anywhere as long as the soil those herbs are in is fertile and well drained. In a container, a raised garden bed, a non-treated pallet, in a windowsill, on a countertop, in a greenhouse, or among your regular garden plants—herbs will go wherever you go, as long as it's not Antarctica.

Container Gardening

When I first started my herb garden, I started in containers on my back deck. Bizarre, I know. But was it really? You might be reading this and thinking this entire garden and soil-building thing is just way too advanced for you right now. I promise, it isn't. Maybe you just want to experiment with herbs before taking on an entire garden. Or maybe you

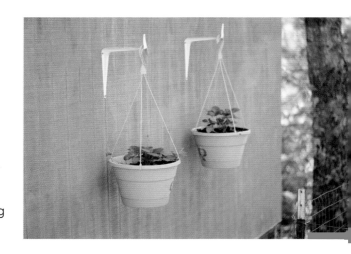

have severe space limitations, like I did, and wonder how you can create healthy soil within containers. Is it even possible to have an herb garden without having a large space? *It's absolutely possible.*

First, you'll need that rich and healthy soil we were talking about a few pages back. No matter what, your soil is key to your herb production and harvest. Simply start with a good base in whatever container or area you'd like to garden. Many people live on rooftops or in apartments, and that's okay! Find a good organic soil to put in a flower pot. Start by filling the pot up halfway with your soil. Add in a handful of manure and compost (you can find it at your nearest garden center if you don't have your own), place your plant (or seeds) into the container or planter bed, cover with more organic soil and another handful of compost, water well, and you're done!

Let it drain

No matter which type of pot you choose, make sure it has drainage holes in the bottom of the container.

Container gardening is fabulous for the gardener who wants herbs all year long without having to dry them, or who is limited on space. I enjoy having smaller pots on my kitchen counter so that I can snip rosemary, thyme, and oregano straight from the countertop into a nice pasta dish or herb bread dough. A small countertop herb garden is so much fun during those harsh winter snow days. It's refreshing and fragrant throughout the year. But if I want a larger harvest, especially to preserve, I enjoy the large planter containers. You can purchase extra-large containers from your garden store, use a five-gallon food-grade bucket, or even just a medium-sized flower pot.

Ceramic, terracotta, wood, or plastic containers all work just fine. You can even use pallets when in a pinch, but they will degrade after the first or second year. Plastic tends to get brittle but can still last quite a while if weather protected. If I were to choose, however, I'd stick with ceramic or terracotta. Both are natural and tend not

Best containers for herbs

Terracotta clay flower pots	Ceramic flower pots or planters
Five-gallon buckets	Wooden boxes
Old fabric grocery bags	Rustic wine barrel
Plastic planters	Wooden crate
Old, hollowed-out fallen tree trunks	Galvanized tub

One of the best things about container gardening is that you can move your containers about. If your herbs aren't getting enough sun in the front, you can pick them up and move them right to the back of the house. Chickens getting into the container? No problem—move it to a different location away from those feathered dinos. Want to have herbs right outside your kitchen door? Go ahead and move them from the garden area right to that prime location.

You can move containers with the sun, with the weather, and for personal preference. And better yet, you can bring herbs that don't winterize well indoors for the colder seasons. In the same respect, you can harden off your herbs more easily when they're in containers each spring.

to have anything chemical within them that could leach into your container soil and, ultimately, into your herbs. Plastic, metal, and nonfood-grade five-gallon buckets can leach chemicals into your soil if not taken care of properly or if they aren't BPA-free.

Raised Garden Beds

I love growing herbs in raised garden beds of their own. Herbs—like echinacea, peppermint, and lemon balm—that spread and creep do well in a confined area. While they may eventually flow over your raised garden bed, they are more easily contained and maintained in a raised bed.

The good and bad of container gardening

THE PROS:

Easily moveable

Perfect for small spaces

Great to have indoors

Produces well with limited space

Allows you to experiment with new herbs

THE CONS:

Doesn't produce as much as herbs in the ground

Will generally have to be replaced every few years

May not thrive with placement of indoor or outdoor conditions

Can be a little costly to get started

Raised beds are a lot like container gardening, except the root system of your plant is allowed to roam freely. There is no stopping point. This means you'll get more herb production in a raised bed than in containers.

With that said, raised beds can be labor intensive to build, and the materials can be costly.

The same soil richness is key, but in a raised bed you don't have to worry about nearly as much weeding. In fact, a raised bed is the best way to implement the no-till method of gardening. You're simply going to layer your soil, compost, manure, and mulch. Voilà! You have a beautiful raised garden bed with rich soil.

When building your raised garden bed, be sure to build it with a wood that won't rot or deteriorate quickly. You can use yellow pine, which naturally holds up to

The dirt on pressure-treated wood

Pressure-treated residential lumber doesn't have to be avoided, but if you're going for "organic" status, it's best to stay away from it. In 2003, the Environmental Protection Agency (EPA) banned the sale of lumber treated with chromated copper arsenate (CCA) for residential use and replaced it with an alternative "safer" treatment. The alternative still leaches slightly into the soil. Typically, all of the treatment is gone after the first year of gardening. But you should still be prepared for these boards to deteriorate after the second or third year.

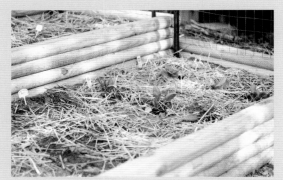

USE THESE ALTERNATIVES:

Yellow pine

Galvanized steel

Water trough

Cinder blocks

Raised bed kits

moisture and pests. You can also use what makes itself available to you through nature, like smaller fallen tree trunks and limbs.

Vertical Gardening

Vertical gardening doesn't work as well with herbs as it does with vegetables, but it is still absolutely attainable. You can purchase vertical containers that can be stacked and planted. You can also create a vertical-type herb garden by using a pallet. However, many vertical gardens don't have much of a soil base, so herb production is typically small compared to large containers and garden plantings that allow the plant to build up a healthier root system.

Planting Herbs among Your Vegetables

I really enjoy planting my herbs in my vegetable garden—it's my preferred method. This is the best option for me in this particular season of life. When you have a farmer-boy running around, dogs chasing after squirrels, and a cow needing to be milked, you like life simplified. It allows me to have all of my plants in one area. It also allows me to plant herbs in places that enhance my vegetables—we call this companion planting (which we'll discuss later).

Better yet, I don't have to replant most of the cold-hearty herbs, and they come back bigger and better each and every year. Herbs like lavender, rosemary, lemon balm, peppermint, thyme, oregano, and echinacea are perennials and will come back each year unless you suffer an apocalyptic winter or have rodents eat your root systems.

If you choose to plant among your regular garden, you'll need to keep space limitations in mind. Each year your herbs are going to come back bigger, wider, and much better than the previous year. Make sure you're planting them along the

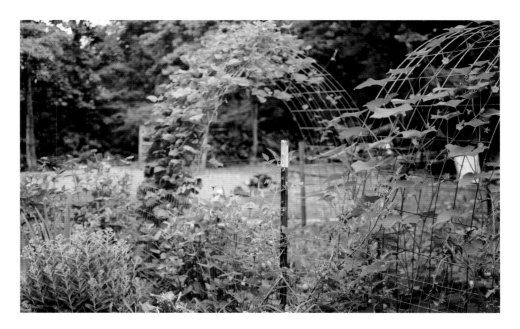

outer edges of your garden, or in areas where you're not hoping to plant those collard greens come fall and then find yourself with no space! Don't ask me how I know this. I just do, okay?

THE WHEN, WHERE, WHY, AND HOW

I have failed at growing herbs so many times, I'd argue whether I'm even the right person to write a book like this. But I feel like because I've failed so many times, it means I've learned how *not* to do it just as much as how to do it.

The very first garden bed that I ever created was a complete disaster. I grew it in my very rocky backyard, right on top of my drainage field. Big ol' stinky fail, my friend. But I was hopeful that I had created a garden completely from scratch with my own two soft little hands. For the first few weeks it thrived. But then, about a month later, it basically just died. Gone. Adíos, amigo. The weeds took over, six cucumbers grew, and I'm pretty sure the mint I tried to grow never made it into the ground. I couldn't even find it. *I still wonder what happened to that mint.*

Let's just be real here. Most days I have absolutely no idea what I'm doing. But that simply means I'm a blank slate, ready and eager to allow nature to show me how it works. I often tell people that their first two to three years of gardening won't amount to anything. They *will* fail. But if they stick with it, the dirt will seep into the pores of their hands with each and every seed they plant, and they will eventually become one with the ground and learn how to grow an efficient garden.

Gardening, to me, is a lot like baking bread. You can give everyone the same recipe, but each person will have a different outcome because their techniques are different. Some will fail miserably and need to practice ten times before they become successful. Others will instantaneously understand and learn. Whichever type of person you are, embrace it.

I could sit here and tell you (and I'm going to) that you have to start your herb seeds in mid- to late winter so that your plants are ready to plant in the spring, but the honest truth is that you could most likely go outside, and throw herb seeds into your fertile soil at the end of fall, and cover them up with some mulch, and those seeds would sprout right up at the exact time they're supposed to. Nature never ceases to amaze me.

But since I don't rely completely on nature, and since our weather is so unpredictable in these parts, I like transplanting my herbs from seed startings. Herbs aren't like peas or green beans that can just be planted in the ground and up they sprout ten days later. They have to be nurtured a bit along the way. True, there are some herbs that you can absolutely and unfailingly throw into the ground and they will grow. Most of the time, they are wild herbs like St. John's wort and milk thistle. These are herbs that grow very naturally in the wild to begin with. But for the necessities, I haven't quite yet given up the reins to nature. And in most climates, you're better off starting your herbs indoors or purchasing them as transplants from your local nursery or farmers' co-op.

WHEN TO START HERBS

Every single region of the country has a hardiness zone. You'll need to see which hardiness zone you're located in before planting (see map on page 54).

If you're starting seeds indoors, the general beginning of herb life is in the late winter months when you begin your other seedlings for the garden. **This is usually about 6–8 weeks before your last frost date.** For me, personally, I'm stuck between two different zones, one of them being mountainous and colder, the other being a bit warmer. This is always a challenge for me, but it's just one of the many luxuries of living in the foothills of a mountain range. I wouldn't trade it for the world.

If you're directly sowing your herb seeds into the ground, wait until the danger of frost has passed in the early spring. You can certainly plant your herb seeds into the ground right before the ground freezes in the late fall and cover with a thick layer of straw or mulch. I've had some luck with this method in years past, but starting seeds indoors is always more efficient.

WHERE TO START HERBS

You'll have several options for where to start your seeds. You'll need to begin with a good container, like a peat moss biodegradable container or a plastic 2- to 4-inch container. You can also plant your herbs in soil blocks, though I find the containers do just as well.

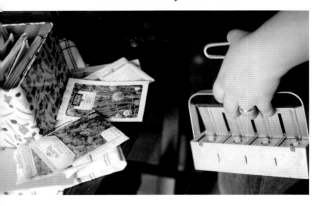

I like to begin my herbs in a small indoor greenhouse. My personal greenhouse is just made of metal tubing and a plastic covering with five racks that I got from my local farm store. The bonus is that this greenhouse, when open in the summer, can act as a drying rack for herbs. It is well worth the small investment.

Because the winter daylight isn't as strong, and also because we heat strictly by wood, a small indoor greenhouse in front of a window that receives good light most of the day is essential. My indoor greenhouse is on wheels and takes up very little space. This allows me to move it about with the sun during the day. However, **if you don't have ample sunlight,** grow lights may be needed for your herb starts.

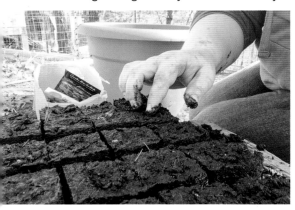

Starting your seeds inside an indoor greenhouse also allows you a better and more efficient experience when hardening off your plants in the spring. You can take the entire greenhouse outside to harden off your plants instead of taking the plants out one by one.

Indoor greenhouses generate heat and capture sunlight, causing your herb starts to flourish more quickly and to be less leggy. When plants become leggy, it means they are stretching super high to reach a light source for more heat and light, therefore producing a less-productive plant.

If you don't wish to use a greenhouse, you can simply place your newly planted herbs in front of a window. Covering them with plastic wrap for the first few days allows the seeds to germinate more quickly, keeps the moisture in, and creates a greenhouse-like effect. Eventually, the plastic will need to come off, but the longer you can keep it on, the better. It creates a mini-permaculture environment while your seeds grow.

Be sure not to overwater your seedlings but maintain a moist soil through the entire germination process.

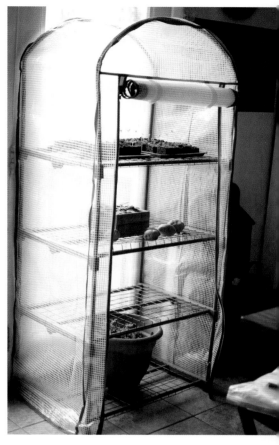

HOW TO START HERBS

Ah ha! Now we're at the real beginning of the art of herbalism. You actually get to do something! You actually have to plant these tiny little seeds into the soil and hope super hard that they grow. You get to nurture them, love them, and play classical music for them. Not really, though I read somewhere years ago that if you play classical music to your plants, they grow better. I don't know if the plants enjoyed it, but I sure did. It was a slight culture shock when I went back to my country tunes.

Don't worry, the process is pretty painless. The seed starting, that is. **Be prepared to lose a few seedlings.** Not all seeds germinate—let's just get that out

The ultimate potting mix

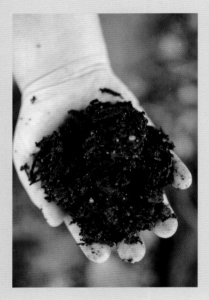

Use this mix to place in your pots when starting seeds indoors.

6 parts compost

3 parts soil (any soil from your property, or bagged soil)

1 part sand

1 part manure (rabbit or store bought)

1 part peat moss

Mix together in a large trash can or container outdoors. Use as needed. When you're ready to transplant your new seedlings into bigger pots, add some bone meal to the individual pots.

there. This is just real life. If you can brace yourself now, you won't feel like much of a failure later.

Planting Seeds

You're going to begin by starting your seedlings 6–8 weeks before your last frost date, sometimes even sooner. For the sake of sanity, let's break this down step by step.

Step 1: Choose your container

I like to begin with a 4-inch container. A peat moss or plastic container works great. You can even repurpose Styrofoam or plastic cups. Just make sure all containers have holes in the bottom for good drainage.

Step 2: Add your dirt

Add your potting mix (like the Ultimate Potting Mix recipe on page 70)[into the planter container, about three-quarters of the way. Place two seeds into your cup (spaced out). Sprinkle a thin layer of soil over the seeds and press lightly.

Step 3: Make a greenhouse

Now that your seeds are planted, cover your containers with plastic wrap or place them in your indoor greenhouse. Covering your containers with plastic wrap will generate a greenhouse-like effect if you don't have a greenhouse available to you. It traps moisture and warms the soil in the container.

Step 4: Give them sunlight

Place your containers in a tray (baking sheets work!) next to a window that gets direct sunlight during the day. You can move your containers with the sun if necessary. If you don't have good sunlight in your home, you'll need to invest in grow lights.

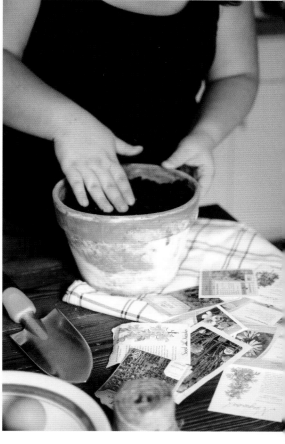

Step 5: Water those babies

Keep your soil moist, but never overwater. Water directly from the bottom of the container by filling your tray with water and allowing your soil to soak up the water naturally from the drainage holes. This cuts back on mold and mildew issues, and also mimics nature, allowing your root system to grow stronger. Your herbs will begin to peek their little green heads out of the soil in 1–2 weeks.

Directly Sowing Seeds

If you're directly sowing your seeds into the ground, you'll need to wait until the danger of frost has passed. As mentioned before, you can absolutely toss some seeds into the ground and cover them heavily in the late fall or early spring with mulch or straw. Just remember to pull back the thick layer of straw that you put over it once the weather begins to even out. For seeds that can be sown directly into the soil in the spring months, the concept is slightly the same.

Step 1:

Make sure your soil is fertile and ready to be planted into. Loose or freshly tilled soil is best.

Step 2:

With a stick or garden tool, draw a line for your rows in the dirt. If you're just randomly sowing into the dirt, you can sprinkle the seeds over the ground space you've chosen.

Step 3:

Add your seeds to the dirt, leaving little spaces according to the package instructions. Then, sprinkle a little potting mix or dirt over the area you've just seeded.

Step 4:

Water thoroughly and cover with a thin layer of mulch. Keep soil moist until seeds begin to sprout, then simply water regularly.

The Sprouting Stage

Now that your seeds have sprouted (in 7–14 days), they're going to need a little tender loving care. Continue to keep them warm and moist if you're starting them indoors, always watering from the bottom but never oversaturating. You'll keep them in their containers and in the tray until they begin to become lush and very green with some height to them. Once they are fairly tall (about 4–5 weeks after planting), you'll need to transplant them into a larger container of their own or into the ground. This will, of course, depend on the plants and their hardiness.

Transplanting into a larger container is extremely easy. You'll simply fill up your new, larger container with a bit of dirt, take your transplant out of its original container, gently break apart some of the root system at the bottom, place it in the new container, and cover with your rich soil. That's it. Water well. And the cycle continues.

Patience is a virtue through the monotony. In about 3-6 more weeks, you'll be transplanting them into your garden.

Hardening Off Your Herbs

Once you're ready to transplant your herbs into the ground or into an outdoor container of your choosing, you'll need to harden off your herbs. Contrary to my firm belief when I first began this journey, you cannot, under any circumstance, just put your brand new, precious herbs right out into the springtime air without hardening them off. It would be like taking a hot shower and then jumping out into the snow. Maybe not as dramatic, but you'd better believe things will begin to, well, tighten up.

It's the same with any plant that has been grown in a greenhouse or indoors for a period of time. Your herb will need to acclimate to the weather before living outdoors for good.

You'll begin the hardening off process by setting your plants out each morning and bringing them in after a couple of hours. As each day progresses, you'll leave them out a little longer, and a little longer, until finally, after about 7-10 days, your plants should be ready to leave outside on their own after the danger of frost has passed.

This is probably the time when you'll feel like a parent to these seedlings. You've done all the growing work, now will they survive the first step of being on their own?

During this process, be sure not to scorch your herbs in the sunshine. Some herbs, like cilantro and thyme, will dry out quickly in the hot spring sun.

The Final Transplant into the Garden

Once your plants are hardened off, you can plant them in their forever home, whether it's your garden or a container of your choosing. I won't lie, this isn't something I learned through trial and error. This is something my husband, the almighty professional landscaper and property maintainer, taught me. We can do this in just a few easy steps.

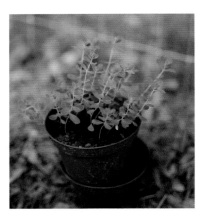

Step 1:

Dig a hole into your soil that is slightly deeper and wider than your transplant (container height). Into the hole, add a small handful of compost/manure mixture.

Step 2:

Take your herb transplant out of its container and gently break apart some of the root system at the very bottom of the plant. This allows the roots to learn how to grow outward instead of continuing to grow in a cylinder-like shape. Place your plant into the hole, cover with your soil, and press down lightly to make sure all of the dirt begins to settle.

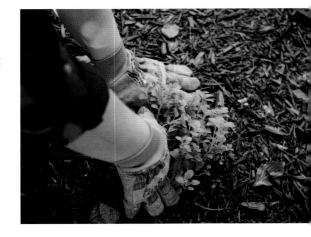

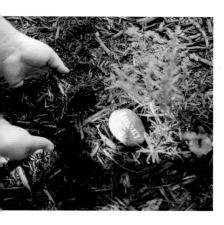

Step 3:

Once you've covered your transplant with soil, add your compost/manure mixture around the base of the plant on top of the soil. Water thoroughly. Don't forget to add your layer of mulch around the base of the plant!

Step 4:

Water thoroughly after transplanting and make sure your soil remains moist for the next few days afterwards, but don't overwater.

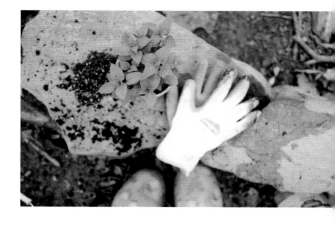

That's it! You've officially planted an herb from start to finish! Don't hate me when I tell you that I tend to just purchase a lot of herbs each year at my local farm store if I need a replacement plant or am just too behind on seed starting. But darn, don't you feel good about yourself now that you know how to grow an herb plant from seed? Also, transplanting an herb from your local farm store involves the same process that I just outlined above. Feeding those herbs in the beginning with good soil and compost and manure really does help produce a more efficient plant and harvest.

FERTILIZING YOUR HERBS

The only time you'll ever need to worry about fertilizing your herbs, or giving them another layer of compost/manure mixture, is right at the beginning or end of the season, and right after a large harvest. When I take large amounts of lavender off of my plants, I always throw down a handful or two of compost and manure for an extra boost of energy and food for each plant. You can also use comfrey tea (see page 28).

WINTERIZING YOUR HERBS

Tender perennial and annual herbs can be brought indoors to winterize through the colder months. This is when container gardening becomes beneficial. Otherwise, you'll lose herbs that are tender to harsh frosts and snow, and your annuals will most certainly not make it through the winter. Some herbs, like basil and parsley, can be winterized indoors to extend their life. Otherwise, you can plant new tender herbs in the fall for a small indoor kitchen herb garden and replant them in the spring outdoors.

There are three different types of herbs when it comes to life cycle—*perennial, annual,* and *biennial.* Knowing these three different types will help you determine whether or not you should try to winterize certain herbs indoors, outdoors (by covering with garden cloth or mulch, or nothing), or by simply replanting the following year.

The easiest countertop herbs for winter

Basil

Oregano

Peppermint

Rosemary

Thyme

Parsley

Chives

Sage

Tarragon

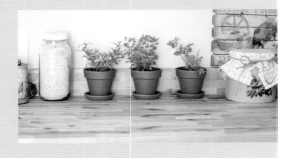

Perennial herbs are herbs that come back every single year. This typically means that they reseed nicely and can reproduce from their original roots. Herbs like peppermint, and especially wild herbs, are famous perennials. Cut these herbs down to about 4–6 inches in height and overwinter outdoors. If you live in an extremely cold region, you'll benefit from adding a thick layer of straw or mulch over your perennial herbs after the first couple of frosts. Other examples of hardy perennials are thyme, sage, fennel, chives, peppermint, echinacea, St. John's wort, and oregano.

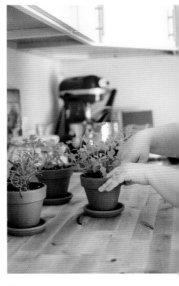

More tender perennials, such as rosemary and marjoram, will need to be cut down just about to the ground to winterize outdoors if they have any chance of coming back and producing the following year. They will also benefit from a good layer of thick straw or mulch after the first few hard frosts. When new growth begins to emerge in the spring, pull back your straw and mulch covering to allow better airflow and sunlight to the plant. When in doubt, rosemary and some tender perennials may have to be brought indoors. You'll need to refer to your zone map before making that final decision.

Annual herbs are ones that will most likely need to be planted every single year. They could reseed themselves, but it is highly unlikely. These herbs can be winterized indoors to prolong their life cycle, but ultimately, they are one-year growers. Basil, cilantro, and dill are great examples of this. You can simply dig the plant up and winterize indoors, knowing that you'll still, more than likely, need to replant a new plant in the spring. Or you can simply cut them down and clean them out at the end of the season after they've gone to seed. Your other option is to plant new plants in containers in the fall and keep them as part of your indoor kitchen herb garden on your countertop.

Biennial herbs are herbs that come back every other year or so. These herbs typically reseed themselves, or regrow from a hardy root, and may appear to come back every year. However, don't be surprised if they suddenly don't come back one year, and then return the next. You'll treat biennial herbs the very same way you treat your annuals. Or you can leave them be, mulch them over the winter months, and keep them moist throughout the seasons. On years that my biennial herbs don't return, I plant a new plant nearby. This is efficient for the homestead herbalist because your years will alternate and you'll begin to have your biennial herb all year long. However, some biennials won't come back at all, depending on your climate. Examples of some biennial herbs are sage, parsley, and mullein. Echinacea is also sometimes considered a biennial herb.

HERBAL COMPANION PLANTING

Interweaving your herbs into your garden beds is an incredible skill that truly blew my mind when I first learned about gardening. Who knew that planting these beautiful, tasty herbs next to your garden vegetables and plants would produce an incredibly healthy fruit or vegetable?

Companion planting is beneficial to the life cycle of your garden vegetables, fruits, and other herbs. You can deter pests or attract helpful insects. Companion planting can also allow the herbs to increase the essential oils that are within other herbs around them. On the other hand, there are some herbs that shouldn't be planted near certain plants. But for the most part, plants just love the heck out of each other.

Almost any herb can be companion planted throughout your garden; however, here are some of the main herbs that I companion plant on a regular basis.

Basil: It's common knowledge that basil pairs well with tomatoes. I'll prepare a plate of homegrown tomatoes, basil, and feta or mozzarella any day of the week during the summer months. I'll devour it myself if no one is around to watch me. And then, I'll make another plate for everyone else. Growing basil near tomatoes, asparagus, oregano, and peppers, helps deter unwanted pests like flies and mosquitoes, and enhances the flavor of its companion plants.

Chives: These do great when planted with any other herbs, bringing out and enhancing the natural essential oils in the companion herbs around it. It is also great when planted next to carrots, squash, and tomatoes, as it repels aphids and enhances flavors. Plant chives with peppers, broccoli, cabbage, eggplant, potatoes, strawberries, rhubarb, and kohlrabi for flavor enhancement and overall plant health. Chives have also been known to deter Japanese beetles.

Garlic: I enjoy planting rows of garlic throughout my garden. It does well with just about any vegetable, but it really does enjoy being near leafy vegetables (cabbage, kale, greens), tomatoes, carrots, and beets. Garlic is great to repel unwanted fungus, Japanese beetles, aphids, rabbits, moths, and snails.

Mint: Mint saves my life from cabbage moths—be it peppermint or spearmint. My goodness, I cannot even express to you how much I need any type of mint (especially peppermint) in the garden. Peppermint and spearmint especially do well among cabbage, kale, and other large leafy greens that are susceptible to cabbage moth damage. Mints also deter ants, aphids, flea beetles, and squash bugs. Just keep it away from your chamomile.

Parsley: Asparagus, corn, tomatoes, peppers, onions, and peas all benefit from companion planting with parsley. Parsley attracts butterflies and pollinators to your garden, and is known to repel beetles.

Rosemary: A fabulous herb that also repels the evil cabbage moth and the bean beetle. It's also the arch nemesis of slugs and snails. Plant among beans, peppers, cabbage, kale, sage, and broccoli.

Thyme: Make thyme your friend, no pun intended. Ever since I've included thyme in my herb garden and around much of my vegetable garden, I've seen a decrease in tomato hornworm and cabbage worm. Thyme pairs well with cabbage, potatoes, strawberries, and tomatoes. Thyme also attracts honeybees, and is great for pollinators. When planted near your bee hives, thyme will enhance the flavor of your honey and promote good bee health.

While there are a lot of herbs you can grow in your garden that are beneficial to your health and other plants, there are also a lot of herbs that you can find growing freely in the wild. We encourage wild herbs, like plantain, to grow among our garden plants and in our yard. In the next chapter, I'll go over some of my favorite wild herbs to forage that I also encourage to grow right in my own backyard. Don't worry, if you can't find them in your region, you can grow many of them right in your garden beds.

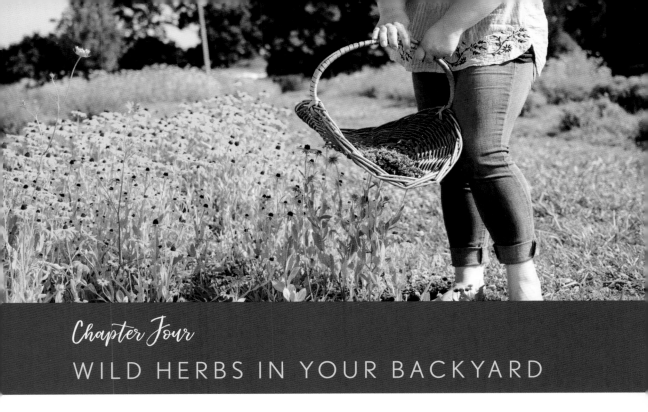

Chapter Four

WILD HERBS IN YOUR BACKYARD

I remember the day my friend invited me to what she called a "crunchy girl" party. I had no idea what that meant, but I was about to find out. I could only hope that we weren't going to be dancing around a fire with herbs in our hair. Fortunately, it was nothing like that.

I introduced myself to about eight other women, grabbed a glass of homemade fermented kombucha, sat down with a plate of quinoa (I had no clue back then that it was pronounced "keen-wa"), and listened. The women talked about herbs, fermentation, natural living, picking wild cress (also known as "creasy greens") from the roadside and making a salad with it. They talked about healing the body from the inside out, raising their livestock naturally, and living life to its fullest.

I heard one of them say "chickens," and immediately my ears perked up. "Chickens? I have chickens!" I blurted out. Finally, something I could connect with. (Isn't that how it always goes, though, when you own chickens?) The women chuckled and then proceeded to ask me about my "crunchiness." People often describe you as "crunchy" when you live a more natural lifestyle than what the rest of society deems normal. Nowadays it looks a lot like eating organic food, raising backyard livestock, eliminating gluten from your diet, and having a passionate love for farmer's markets and natural remedies.

Even though I wasn't quite "crunchy" yet, this meeting with like-minded women set me on a path to living a more natural lifestyle. I wanted to walk through the woods, point at plants, and know what they were. I wanted to pick a leaf and say to someone, "Here, put this on your bee sting. It will heal it." I wanted the knowledge and ability to be confident about what plants were safe and what plants were big no-nos.

Don't pick that roadside herb!

It's great to pick wild herbs on the roadside, but avoid picking them when they are *directly* on the roadside or growing near ditches. You'll do more harm than good to your body because these plants are contaminated with pollutants and chemical sprays.

When your mind begins to realize how many things around you are edible or medicinal, it literally has an awakening. You start looking at the world a lot differently than you did before. Instead of getting rid of that plantain weed in your yard, you now wonder if you can use it for something, like a toothache, a bug bite, or in a soap. Instead of treating your pasture with harsh chemicals, you let the wild herbs grow. And when you see those wild violets come up in your manicured yard, you don't just think of them as pretty weeds anymore. You realize that you can make something with them, something beautiful, like a syrup for iced tea, or a lovely garnish for your salad that's also healthful.

People are going to think you're eccentric, by the way. In today's fast-paced society, a manicured lawn with lush green grass is something many strive for—clearly a "First World" problem. And there's really nothing wrong with that . . . until there is. Whenever I see someone killing the weeds in their yard, I cringe a little.

It's a stark reminder of just how far removed we are from a generation of people who knew that everything had a purpose.

That wild herb could be the thing that cures your child's infection from a cut in his foot. It could be the very thing your milk cow needs to help boost her production or give her much-needed energy. In fact, if we let more wild herbs grow and learned how to use them correctly, we could have our own free pharmacy right in our own backyard.

There are hundreds upon hundreds of wild herbs that I could share with you, but I'll focus on my favorites and some of the most common and easily identified.

MY TOP WILD HERBS

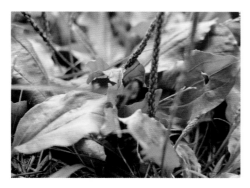

Plantain

Botanical Name: *Plantago lanceolata*

Family: Plantaginaceae

Common Name(s): greater plantain, broadleaf plantain

Perennial growth

Parts used: leaves

Uses: astringent, expectorant, stops bleeding, soothes skin, anti-inflammatory, soothes cough, treats bee stings , protects liver, treats kidney stones

Harvest: Harvest leaves at maturity all season long.

History: Plantain is one of those weeds that will grow just about anywhere—in a sidewalk crack, in the yard, along roadsides. Native Americans used to call it "white man's foot" because it seemed to follow the pathways of the early settlers. The Saxons considered it as one of their nine sacred herbs. And in early Christianity, it was seen as a symbol of Christ, as the weed would follow the well-trodden pathway of the multitudes that followed after Him.

We know today that this weed popped up in all of these places because it grows in areas that most things will not. It thrives along roadsides, and even in gravel.

Plantain can be used internally and externally, though it is most often used externally. Use plantain in cough syrups to bring relief and to soothe the throat. Apply the plant topically to relieve skin irritation, burns, bug bites, bee stings, and eczema.

It has also been known to soothe toothaches by chewing on the leaves.

How We Use It: Plantain is probably my favorite wild herb. I use it on bee stings, in salves and balms, to give to my livestock as a natural anti-inflammatory, and during bouts of sore throat.

Safety and Dosage: There are no known precautions or safety issues with plantain.

For a standard 1:5 tincture, take 7 mL up to three times a day.

2–3 teaspoons of dried plantain can be consumed in a tea.

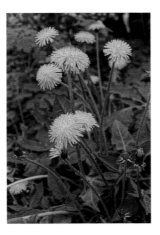

Dandelion

Botanical Name: *Taraxacom officinale*

Family: Asteraceae

Common Name(s): lion's tooth

Perennial growth

Parts used: leaves and roots, sometimes flowers

Uses: diuretic, appetite stimulant, digestive bitter, mild laxative, lymphatic cleansing, supports liver function, reduces eczema, regulates intestinal flora, detoxifies

Harvest: Harvest root after dandelion flower head opens. Harvest leaves and flower heads all season long.

History: Native Americans considered dandelions to be a prized culinary herb and edible that helped with the digestive system and in detoxifying the body. They used them in poultices for skin irritations and wounds, and they often chewed on the root for tooth pain.

Today, we use dandelions to detoxify the body and lymphatic system. They can be used to support healthy liver function and can be eaten in salads and other dishes. There is so much to be praised when it comes to the dandelion. Who knew such an amazing weed could hold such incredible benefits?

How We Use It: Chickens and livestock love dandelions, and so do we. Use the leaves in salads, much like kale, as a healthy way to regulate gut flora. Use the heads, leaves, and root for medicinal uses like tinctures and teas.

Safety and Dosage: Do not take internally if you have gallstones or when you have an obstruction in your digestive tract.

Dandelions can be eaten liberally.

A 1:5 tincture can be taken with a dose of 10–15 drops up to three times per day as needed.

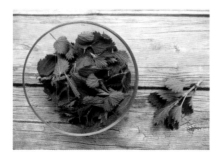

Stinging Nettle

Botanical Name: *Urtica dioica*

Family: Urticaceae

Common Name(s): nettle

Perennial growth

Parts used: leaves, roots

Uses: astringent, diuretic, stops bleeding, detoxifies, soothes urinary tract, soothes asthma

Harvest: Stinging nettle should be harvested in the spring, right before the flowers bloom, for the most potent medicinal value. However, it can be harvested all year long.

History: Stinging nettle has been used throughout history for various purposes. It can be made into cloth or twine, and it can be used medicinally as well.

Nettle was one of the nine powerful herbs that the Saxons used and valued, and it was thought to combat evil spirits.

How We Use It: Today, we use it in tonics, teas, and tinctures for various ailments, and it offers a grand amount of vitamin C. You can eat stinging nettle after steaming it, and use it much like you would spinach.

Some speculate that the plant can stimulate hair growth, although that hasn't been proven.

Nettle can also be used to bring relief to arthritis and painful joints when used externally in a salve or internally in a tincture.

Safety and Dosage: There are no known precautions with nettle, however, it can cause a numbing or tingling effect when it comes into contact with skin. In rare cases, some people have developed severe rashes when touching nettle directly. When in doubt, use caution and wear gloves when harvesting and handling nettle.

A 1:5 tincture can be taken by mouth in 20–30 drops as needed, up to three times a day.

Steep 2–3 teaspoons nettle root or dried leaves to make an infused tea.

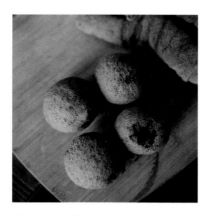

Black Walnut Hull

Botanical Name: *Juglans nigra*

Family: Juglandaceae

Perennial growth

Parts used: powdered hull

Uses: anti-inflammatory, antiparasitic, antioxidant, antifungal, protects nerve cells, improves cardiovascular health

Harvest: Dry out the casings of the hulls of the walnuts either from the tree or once they've fallen on the ground, then grind down into powder.

How to dry walnut hulls

Walnut hulls can be a bit difficult to dry, but with a little patience the outcome is worth the wait.

Start by cleaning off your walnut hulls from the walnut, making sure you use gloves! The black from the hulls will stain your hands for weeks. Next break the hulls into pieces as small as possible. Allow them to sit out in the sun or in a sunny window for several days. The hulls will become completely black and will feel leathery when handled. Once they reach the leathery stage, grind the hulls into a fine powder in a coffee grinder or food processor. Lay the powder onto a cookie sheet and allow to dry for another few days. Once completely dry, store in an airtight container in a cool, dry place.

History: Most people don't think of a walnut hull as an herb, but it absolutely has medicinal properties.

Walnut hulls have been used extensively as a dye and for face paint in tribal cultures. In fact, if you don't wear gloves when shelling walnuts, your hands will be black for days, sometimes lasting more than a week.

Herbalist Nicholas Culpeper prescribed walnut hulls to draw out venom from spider bites and snake venom in the first century AD. Native Americans would use them to treat skin conditions, and as a mosquito repellent. They were also used as a natural laxative.

Today we use black walnut hulls for their antibacterial and antiparasitic properties, especially in livestock. They are also still used as a natural laxative.

How We Use It: You'll find black walnut hulls in almost all of my antiparasitic and antibacterial tinctures. It is an aggressive herb that should be respected but used more often than it is!

Safety and Dosage: Black walnut hulls shouldn't be used for extended periods of time. If you have a nut allergy, black walnut hulls can cause skin irritation and allergic reactions. Do not take any other medications until two hours after taking black walnut hull as it can counteract them.

1 teaspoon of the powder can be taken in a tea infusion up to three times per week.

Ten drops of a 1:5 tincture can be taken up to two times a day for no more than two weeks.

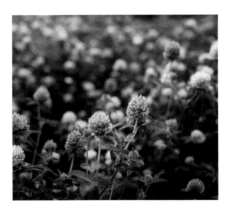

Red Clover

Botanical Name: *Trifolium pratense*

Family: Fabaceae

Common Name(s): clover, red clover

Perennial growth

Parts used: leaves and flowers

Uses: balances hormones and menopause, treats and prevents osteoporosis

Harvest: Harvest clover tops and leaves as needed.

History: Red clover has been planted in pastures and used for livestock feed for years. It is a great cover crop, and it also promotes good fertility and reproductive health in animals.

Today, we use red clover to help promote progesterone and balance estrogen in women. Menopausal women will especially benefit from red clover, as it balances the hormones and treats and prevents osteoporosis, evening out bone density.

How We Use It: We use red clover strictly as a livestock herb. Give this herb to mothers and potential mothers to help their reproductive systems and to balance out hormones.

This is also an herb I give to friends and family who are dealing with hormone imbalance and menopause.

Safety and Dosage: Consult your doctor before taking if you are using hormone replacement therapy. Do not take while taking blood thinners.

A tea of 1 teaspoon dried clover to 8 ounces of water up to three times per day can be taken as a tea infusion.

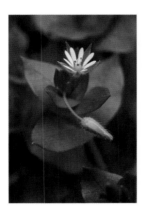

Chickweed

Botanical Name: *Stellaria media*

Family: Caryophyllaceae

Common Name(s): chickweed

Perennial growth

Parts used: leaves and stems

Uses: detoxifies, anti-inflammatory, antibacterial, restores nutrients

Harvest: Chickweed can be harvested all year long as it is available, as long as the leaves are still bright and green.

History: Chickweed will grow just about anywhere. It's joked that it even grows in Antarctica, but we all know that's not true. There isn't a whole lot of history or information about chickweed, but we do know that it has offered medicinal benefits throughout the centuries and is even used in modern day folk medicine.

How We Use It: We typically use chickweed as an external component to heal and cleanse wounds, rashes, infections, and other areas of the body.

Chickweed is great for adding to your salads, and for your livestock.

Safety and Dosage: There are no known precautions with chickweed.

Use in external preparations like salves and ointments.

Can be eaten in salads for nutritional value and benefits.

Take a 1:5 tincture of 30 drops as needed.

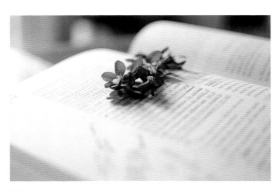

Wild Violet

Botanical Name: *Viola odorata*

Family: Violaceae

Common Name(s): wild violet, sweet violet

Perennial growth

Parts used: flowers and leaves

Uses: antiseptic, expectorant, helps reduce cough, diuretic

Harvest: Wild violet flower tops should be harvested at peak maturity and color. Leaves, however, can be harvested all season long.

History: Wild violets have been used in perfumes, as dyes, to flavor teas and syrups, and in "love potions."

Today, we utilize this herb for its ability to boost vitamin A and C, to relieve coughs, and as a diuretic.

How We Use It: I love collecting wild violets in my backyard and around the farm during the spring months. We make violet syrup mainly for its taste and add it to flavor teas and breads. You can find this recipe on page 130.

Safety and Dosage: There are no known precautions or safety issues with wild violets.

Use 2–3 tsp of dried leaves in a tea infusion.

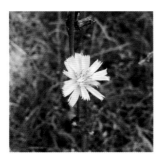

Chicory

Botanical Name: *Cichorium intybus*

Family: Asteraceae

Common Name(s): chicory, kasni

Perennial growth

Parts used: roots and leaves

Uses: diuretic, coffee substitute, antioxidant, aids in digestion, stimulates appetite, releases gallstones

Harvest: Harvest leaves throughout the season, harvest mature root from March through May.

History: Chicory lines the roadside here in the Virginia countryside, but you'll only see its purple flowers in the morning, or when the weather is cooler. Once afternoon hits and the sun is at its warmest, the flowers close up to protect themselves. It's quite a sight to see!

Historically, chicory was widely used as an alternative to coffee in many countries. It also aids in digestion and helps detoxify the body.

How We Use It: We enjoy using chicory as treats for our livestock at times (root), and chicory adds a great hazelnutty taste to coffee (or can be used as a substitute for coffee).

Safety and Dosage: There are no known safety precautions with chicory.

Boil 1 teaspoon of dried root in 1 cup of water to create a decoction tea. Drink 1–1½ cups per day as needed.

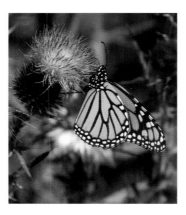

Milk Thistle

Botanical Name: *Silybum marianum*

Family: Asteraceae

Common Name(s): Mary's thistle

Perennial growth

Parts used: seeds

Uses: promotes good liver function, detoxifies liver, gallbladder health, spleen health

Harvest: Milk thistle seeds can be harvested at the end of the season by pulling off the flower head into a brown paper bag.

History: The ancient Greeks and Romans used milk thistle for quite a few ailments, though not all are relevant today. They would often soothe bites and stings with milk thistle, no doubt because it was widely available in fields.

We often see an abundance of milk thistle in fields that have been overgrazed or are not as nutrient-rich as they could be. Milk thistle, like many wild herbs, thrives in less-than-ideal conditions.

Today, we use milk thistle to protect, heal, and detoxify the liver, gallbladder, and spleen—with emphasis on the liver. It has been known to rejuvenate the liver of those affected by alcohol and hepatitis. It can be given to patients who are taking chemotherapy to help protect the liver. It's also widely used along with over-the-counter medicines, like pain killers, that could harm your internal organs.

How We Use It: Milk thistle is a new herb to our homestead, but it has quickly become one of my favorites. We use milk thistle whenever we take an over-the-counter pain killer. Down goes the pain killer, and alongside it, a capsule of milk thistle seed powder to help protect our livers and other internal organs, and to allow our bodies to process medications effectively and naturally.

Safety and Dosage: There are no known safety precautions with milk thistle.

In a 1:5 tincture, 30 drops three times a day can be taken as needed.

Powdered milk thistle can be taken in 1–2 capsules daily as needed or as a preventative.

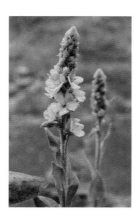

Mullein

Botanical Name: *Verbascum* spp.

Family: Scrophulariaceae

Common Name(s): Aaron's rod

Biennial growth

Parts used: leaves and flowers

Uses: sedative, diuretic, expectorant, astringent, anti-inflammatory, softens skin, aids in upper respiratory relief

Harvest: Mullein is found on roadsides and in fields. Harvest when plant is mature and in areas free of pollutants. Harvest the large leaves that are closest to the ground throughout the season. Summer flowers can be collected in early morning.

History: The Greek physician Dioscorides was one of the first to talk about mullein, and he used it for lung conditions. The Romans also used it for the same reason, as well as for a natural dye. American folklore and herb history is sprinkled with accounts of the properties of mullein.

How We Use It: Use this herb for lung and upper respiratory conditions. Use it as a poultice for cuts and swollen glands to cleanse the wound. Use it as a natural sedative and to reduce inflammation. It can also be used in salves, lotions, and ointments to help heal and soothe the skin.

Safety and Dosage: Be sure to get rid of the small hairs on the mullein leaf before using internally, as it can cause irritation to the mouth and throat. Otherwise, there are no known safety precautions.

In a 1:5 tincture, take 30 drops three times a day as needed.

Make a tea using 1–3 teaspoons of dried mullein.

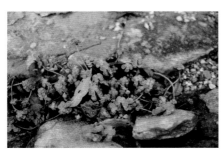

Purslane

Botanical Name: *Portulaca oleracea*

Family: Portulacaceae

Common Name(s): Common purslane, little hogweed, parsley, red root, verdolaga, duckweed, fatweed

Annual growth

Parts used: leaves and stems

Uses: mostly used in culinary dishes, but can also be used to help soothe insect bites and stings

Harvest: Harvest in the early morning before the sun is too harsh during the day. Cut stems right at ground level without disturbing the root system. Wash thoroughly.

History: Often seen as a nuisance plant in the garden or yard, purslane has received a bad reputation for decades. But with the expansion of modern day gardeners, and the popularity of the internet, we've discovered that purslane isn't any different than watercress or spinach. In fact, it has an equal amount of nutritional benefits.

Purslane is one of few plants that has been proven to grow all over the world. From the Middle East and Europe to North and South America, purslane simply grows everywhere, dating all the way back to the seventh century BC.

How We Use It: Today, you can find purslane growing in your garden and backyard. It even adapts to living in the cracks of sidewalks and stone walls. But don't expect to see purslane popping up until the soil remains warm throughout late spring, as purslane really thrives on sunlight, warmth, and well-moistened soil.

Purslane will naturally reseed itself each year. However, you can also purchase seeds to encourage natural growth on your property. Just make sure you put it in an area that you're willing to share! It can spread quickly.

Throw purslane stems and leaves into salads or cook it down the same way you would spinach in other culinary dishes. You can even create a pesto out of purslane.

In a pinch, you can use crushed, fresh purslane on insect bites and stings to help soothe the skin, but that's about the extent of its medicinal uses.

Safety and Dosage: There are no known precautions with purslane; however, it has not yet been proven safe to eat when pregnant. Please use caution.

Yarrow

See "The Homesteader's Herb List" (chapter 2).

Elderberry

See "The Homesteader's Herb List" (chapter 2).

IDENTIFYING YOUR WILD HERBS

It's extremely important to be confident in your ability to know which wild herbs are usable and which ones you should stay away from. It's easy, for example, to confuse Queen Anne's lace with poison hemlock. Both have similar-looking flower patterns and leaves. But the smallest amount of poison hemlock, when ingested, can be fatal. The more you get to know wild herbs, the more you'll notice that Queen Anne's lace has a hairy stem, while poison hemlock's is smooth with purple blotches.

You also can't always assume that everything in your field is good for you or your livestock. There are things in and around your pasture that could potentially harm your animals or you. It's beneficial to get to know not just a plant's appearance as a whole, but its individual parts—flower, stem, leaves—as well.

MATERIA MEDICA JOURNALING

In the world of herbalism, the information about the individual parts of an herb can be found in a materia medica, which is a journaling method used by those who study herbs. Materia medica books give you a list, much like this book, about herbs and how they are used. It lists the botanical name and common name (example: Echinacea's botanical name is *Echinacea purpurea,* but its common name is "Echinacea" or "Purple coneflower"), the parts of the plant that are used, where you can find it, the botanical description, harvesting guidelines, preparations, uses, taste, smell, and dosage of the plant. It also has a photo or illustration of the herb and its many parts.

A materia medica *what?*

I know. I thought *"too much information"* when I first heard about this, but I have since learned that keeping a journal about herbs in my local area, property, and region is really helpful, and I think you'll find it helpful, too.

Consider your materia medica journal very much like a personal reference file for your herbs. Each herb has a profile telling you the name, uses, side effects, and safety information. This journal will be your friend at home *and* in the field.

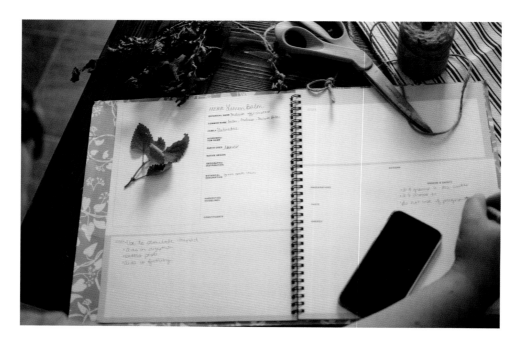

MAKING YOUR MATERIA MEDICA JOURNAL

Making a journal isn't hard at all. You can find printables online, or you can even purchase premade journals that are blank or that include the materia medica outline. Whatever you choose will work just fine. Even a blank sheet of paper is better than nothing. Either way, here are the basics of what needs to be included in your outline.

Herb Identification: Begin with a photo or drawing of the herb. When you're out in the field or foraging in the woods, making a mental note about an herb that you're curious about really isn't good enough. Snap a photo, or carry your journal with you and draw the herb in as much detail as possible, concentrating on the flower, stem, and leaves. This illustration, or photo, will help you identify the herb once you're able to sit down and do some more research.

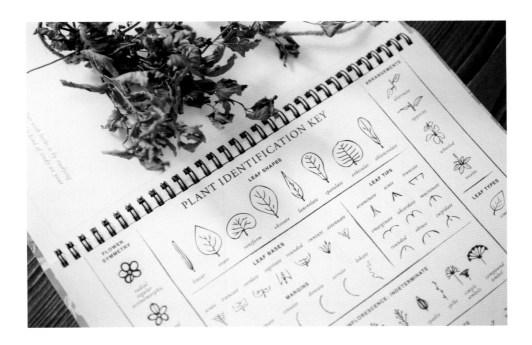

List the Names: Once you're back to a location where you can begin research, you'll need to list the different names of the herb. The botanical name, family name, and common names are all great things that should be added to your journal page. Oftentimes, we call herbs by their common names, not realizing that many things can go by the same name. For example, not all marigold plants are *Calendula* plants. *Calendula* is the botanical name, not the common name. But the same plant can also go by "marigold" or "pot marigold." Always search by botanical name, of course, when looking for the proper medicinal herb. You'll find these names listed in italics beside most common plant names.

Pharmacological Actions and Energetics: Actions of the herb are things that the herb does. For example, is the herb an astringent? A diuretic? The energetics of an herb are descriptions of how the herb interacts with the body and bodily systems. Overall, you're looking for what the herb is traditionally used for.

Description and History: It's really fun to learn about the history of an herb. This allows us to see how people centuries and generations ago used this herb in its natural form. Give a description of how the herb has been used throughout history, and how it is used today.

Indications: Make a list of what the herb can be used for when ingested, used topically, and used aromatically. This is where you'll also list whether an herb is used for a specific purpose or detailed circumstance. It's important to pinpoint, in detail, what an herb can be used for.

Clinical Uses: This is the place where you want to list modern notes, scientifically proven studies, clinical trials, and more. In other words, prove that the herb can do what you say it can do.

Safety and Dosage: This is one of the most important parts of the outline. List the safety precautions and proper dosing amounts of the herb. This is especially true if children or pregnant and nursing mothers should steer clear of this herb.

Side Effects: We always want to know about side effects. Are there any side effects? Could the herb interact with medications, etc.?

Methods of Administration: What parts of the plant can be used? And furthermore, how do you use them? Can you eat it, or is it for external use only? Can you use the entire plant, or just the root? Can you make an infusion, tincture, syrup, or salve?

Similar Herbs and Combinations: We like to combine herbs when creating decoctions (boiled water infusions), salves, soaps, and more. In this section, it's great to list what other herbs make good companions for this specific herb, and it's also a great place to write down herbs that are similar to the one you are journaling. They can be similar in uses, or they can be similar in appearance. You might wish to make a note that even though they appear similar, they have different characteristics. This is also a great place to record wild herbs that look similar but could be potentially harmful (remember me talking about Queen Anne's lace versus poison hemlock?).

Keep this journal with you at all times when you're out in the field, foraging, or even on the road. You never know when you might find a plant that needs identifying! But also, it's just satisfying to learn and expand your knowledge of wild herbs wherever you go. Who knows? You might stumble across something amazing.

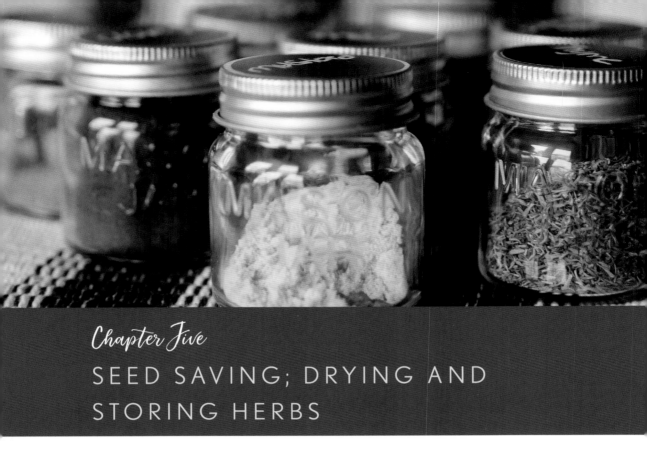

Chapter Five

SEED SAVING; DRYING AND STORING HERBS

Let's talk now about seed saving and storing your herbs, shall we? This task sounds daunting, but it's really quite simple. You've put so much hard work into your harvest, now you'll need to ensure that you've saved and stored it properly. Nothing is worse than finding a moldy jar of dehydrated herbs in the pantry or wilted fresh herbs on the kitchen counter.

Seed saving, properly drying your harvest, and efficiently and safely storing your dried herbs—these are things that must be done no matter what you plan to do with your herbs after they are grown. Technically, you don't *have* to save your seeds. But by doing so, you'll have a better plant that is more adapted to your soil and climate for years to come should you need to plant seeds again the following year.

And drying and storing your herbs safely and properly is something that every herbal homesteader needs to master. Don't worry, it's quite easy, and you have options!

SAVING YOUR SEEDS

Saving your seeds is absolutely painless. It sounds labor intensive, but keep in mind that each new flower head of an herb can hold dozens, even hundreds, of seeds. The most complicated decision is to decide when to allow your herbs to go to seed and when to harvest them.

Many herbs will self-seed, such as calendula and chamomile. This means that the seeds will fall to the ground and grow the following year. You can still harvest seeds from these plants, and I do encourage it just in case there's an awfully wet winter that prevents the plant from self-sowing. I also encourage my herbs to self-seed as much as possible because they always return bigger and better since they know exactly when to pop up out of the ground, and have grown resilient.

Herbs that don't self-sow, or that you want to save seeds from, will need to "go to seed" before you can harvest the seeds. This means that you'll have to allow plants to develop a flower head, which is where your seeds will grow, or you'll have to hold back the bulbs of certain herbs, like garlic and onions, to replant the following year. You can

Seeds I save

Calendula	Chamomile
Echinacea	Garlic (bulbs)
Black-eyed Susan	Onion (bulbs)
Cilantro	Ginseng
Lemon Balm	Cayenne

do this by drying out the bulbs and storing them in a cool place until you're ready to replant. Garlic and onions can be sown in the fall and reaped in the spring, or sown in the spring and reaped in the fall.

Allowing the flower head to stay on the plant as long as possible, so that it dries mostly on its own, is very important. Some plants will drop their seeds before they are completely dry. These seeds will have to be harvested a little "under ripe" and dried indoors. But try your hardest to allow them to dry on the plant itself in order to get the most mature seed possible.

Step 1:

With a brown paper bag or envelope hovering under the flower head of your herb, gently remove the flower head into the bag or envelope. Be sure to harvest seeds from the healthiest and biggest plants. Just as with genetics in animals, genetics in plants make a big difference when reproducing.

Step 2:

Once you've gathered your herb flower heads, you'll need to lay them out on a flat surface indoors, or away from the breeze. As you take each flower head out, you can gently shake it into the bag/envelope so that the seeds are captured. Any seeds that are still in the flower head can be picked out or allowed to dry a little longer indoors.

Step 3:

Some seeds may need to be cleaned. You can do this by rubbing them around in a mesh strainer or sieve, separating the seeds and casings. Lay out on a drying rack, towel, or paper to completely finish drying if necessary. If your seeds still have flower petals on them, remove the petal ends.

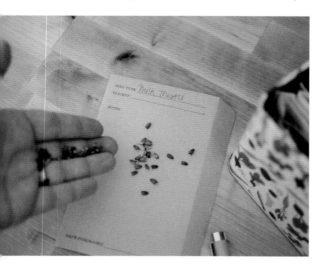

Step 4:

Once the seeds are completely extracted and dried out, store them in a brown paper envelope or an airtight container, being sure to label the name of the herb and the year that you harvested them. Keep them out of sunlight and store in a dry area.

And that's it! You've officially saved your herb seeds for subsequent-year plantings.

I've planted saved seeds that are as much as six years old. Keep in mind that as the seeds age, they can lose their viability. It's best to save new seeds each year or every few years to replenish your supply.

DRYING YOUR HERB HARVEST

Drying herbs is so much fun. My only dilemma is that I often don't have enough room for the harvest that comes in all at once in the summer months. Oftentimes, you'll have more herbs than you need to use at one time. I'm pretty sure my family would fire me if I spent an entire week cooking with only the large basket of oregano that I'd just brought inside. We'd be on oregano overload—so much so that we'd probably start smelling like it. *Is that pizza I smell? Why do you smell like a lasagna?!* I digress, even though I really love oregano and its cute little leaves.

So the option that best suits the homesteader is to preserve the abundant harvest. We can do this in many ways, but it always begins with dehydrating your herbs. This is important because you'll most likely need these herbs throughout the winter and seasons when fresh herbs aren't available.

Before you can create any type of tincture or product with your herbs, it's always best to dry them. Because herbs are a living thing, they retain much of their moisture right after being harvested. It can take days to weeks for them to completely dry out. If not dried properly, the herb can ruin your product due to the moisture buildup. This can cause your remedy to go rancid or have impurities.

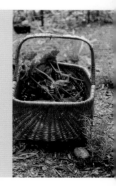

When to harvest

Always harvest your herbs in the morning or late evening. Morning is always preferred. Never harvest herbs midday. Harvesting your herbs in the morning after the dew has dried keeps the natural essential oils in the herb intact. The flavor of the herb is also more potent in the morning.

Mostly, though, we want to dry our own herbs to make teas and meals. There are multiple techniques and ways to do this, including hanging them to dry, drying them in the oven, dehydrating them with a dehydrator, and even laying them out in the sun to dry.

Drying with a dehydrator: Wash your herbs thoroughly, pat dry, and place them on the rack of your dehydrator in a single layer. If the leaves are medium to large, you can remove them from the stem of the herb. If you are dehydrating flowers, remove the flower head from the stem.

Turn your dehydrator to the lowest heat setting possible (between 95°F –125°F). If there is not a heat setting, run the dehydrator for the shortest time possible, checking your leaves periodically. Depending on the herb, it takes between thirty minutes and four hours to dry them in a dehydrator.

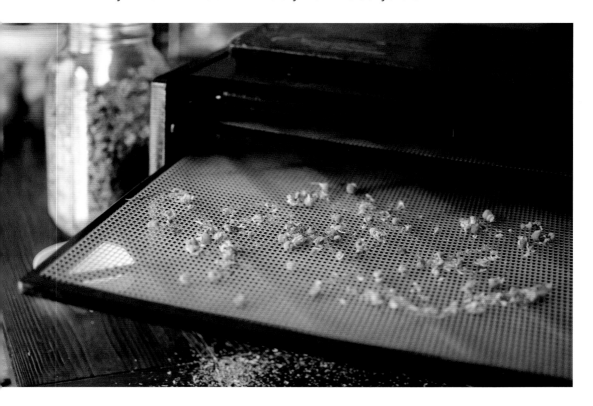

Make your own herb powder

Did you know you can make your own herb powder and salts for cooking and herb products? It's easy!

Herb of choice (garlic and onion are popular)

Dehydrator

Salt (optional)

1. Cut herb into very thin slices, and lay out on dehydrator mats.

2. Dehydrate herbs according to dehydrator instructions for that particular herb until completely dry and crispy.

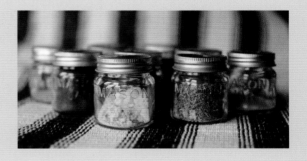

3. Put herbs in a food processor and blend until powdery. Add salt if you'd like, for extra taste!

4. Store in an airtight container for 12–18 months.

Drying with your oven: I was too cheap to purchase a dehydrator when I first started growing my herbs, so instead, I used my oven. I do love my dehydrator now. The oven method is extremely easy, but it can make your house a little warm in the summer.

Simply place your herbs either directly onto the oven rack, on a drying rack (I use a cookie drying rack), or on a cookie sheet.

Set your oven to the lowest setting possible. Mine goes down to 150°F. Make sure it's less than 190°F.

Place your herbs in the oven, leaving your oven door cracked a bit so that the air can flow. I use an old wooden spoon jacked into the top of the oven door. Check on your herbs in fifteen-minute intervals, as they seem to dry more quickly in the oven than in a dehydrator, most likely due to the higher heat. If using a cookie sheet, flip your herbs halfway through the process.

Drying with drying racks and the sun: One of the more common methods for dehydrating herbs is to use drying racks. You can make your own drying racks, or you can purchase them online or from your local farm store. Drying racks are simply racks with slats or mesh wire on the bottom. You place your herbs in a single layer and allow the herbs to dry naturally indoors or outdoors in a protected area. Drying racks are stackable as well.

Obviously, this method can take much longer, sometimes up to a week or more.

You can also place your racks outside in the direct sunlight, not stacked. This makes the drying process much easier. For tender herbs like mint, oregano, and thyme, I simply place them on a rack and set them on my back deck in the direct sunlight for the entire day, moving them with the sun. By the end of the day, I have dried herbs that didn't take much work!

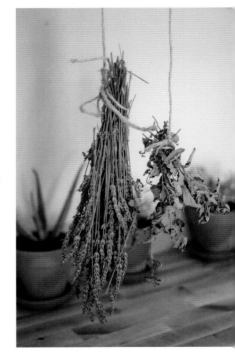

Drying herbs by hanging: The most popular way to dry herbs is to hang them to dry. This is a little more risky, as hanging too thick a bundle can promote lack of airflow, causing your herbs to mold quickly. However, it really is an efficient way to dry herbs that have less moisture content, like thyme, lavender, and chamomile.

Group your herbs in smaller bundles and tie at the very end of the stems with hemp rope or twine. Hang in a sunny window or in an open space in your kitchen, allowing ample airflow through the herbs.

While there are different methods to drying herbs, you'll know when they are dry only by look and touch. They will be crumbly, easily detachable from their stems, and won't feel squishy or look wet. If you see dark-colored spots on the herbs, that typically means they are not yet finished drying. More time is necessary. If your herbs have molded, you will know immediately by the fluffy white stuff on them.

This drying process can, again, take as little as a couple of days to a few weeks, depending on your environment, location, and how thick the bundle is.

STORING DRIED HERBS

Once dry, store your herbs in airtight containers. You can use a vacuum sealer if you wish, but we do not. I like using mason jars with plastic screw-top lids. This allows me to see the herbs quickly, while still keeping them fresh. If you're making something specific with them, like a tea, go ahead and mix the dried herbs into a dry tea mixture. Otherwise, they can remain separate for later use. You can even label your plastic screw-top lids with a permanent marker, as the marker washes away with a little soap.

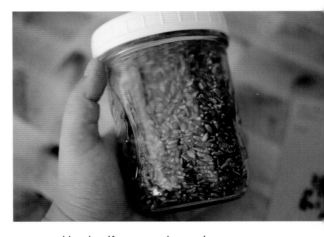

After labeling your storage container, store your dried herbs in a cool, dry, and dark area, such as a pantry that doesn't get sunlight. Sunlight can be detrimental to the shelf life of herbs.

Whole herbs last longer than crushed or processed herbs. If you can keep the herb intact, it will last much longer and prove to be a stronger product for you.

Dried Herb Shelf Life

Dried herbs can last anywhere from six months to three years. It will depend on the herb and the quality of the environment around it. Herbs never technically go bad, but they do begin to lose their potency after the twelve-month mark. If herbs become extremely dull or lose their aroma, toss and replace. Typical replacement shelf life is 12–18 months. This is why I don't recommend keeping large batches of herbs on hand unless you use them daily. Small batches from your garden each year work just fine. Preserve them one step further by making salves, tinctures, and syrups.

STORING FRESH HERBS

Many times I'll hold on to some fresh herbs when I'm drying. I might find that I need them in the next few days or couple of weeks. Depending on the herb, you can efficiently keep them fresh by using a few simple tricks.

Herbs like cilantro and other tender herbs need much more attention than others, but all are about the same. Once you've cut your harvest, place the stems in a jar of water as if you were placing flowers in a vase. Next, cover the tops of the herbs with plastic wrap or a plastic bag, almost making an umbrella or mini greenhouse for your herb tops. This keeps the moisture in your herbs and ensures that the herbs don't dry out or become scorched by the cold air in the fridge. Place the herbs in your refrigerator until you need them.

This method works well for culinary herbs like parsley, cilantro, oregano, chives, and basil. Many times I find herbs like cilantro and parsley can last more than a week in the fridge if covered properly.

For thicker-stemmed herbs like rosemary, thyme, oregano, and sage, you can place them in a wet paper towel and keep them in the refrigerator until ready to use. Check them daily to rewet your towel if necessary. You can also simply place them in a jar of water, again, like flowers in a vase, and let them sit on your countertop.

Once your herbs become dull and extra limp, toss them to the chickens (if you have 'em!) and start all over again.

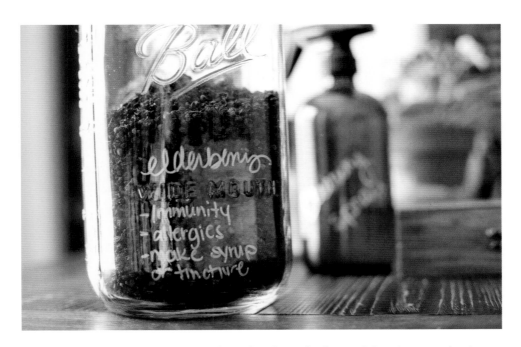

Your stored herbs, whether fresh or dried, can be beautiful and put on display in your pantry or on your countertop. No matter where you choose to put them, the aromatics will certainly be delightful, and you'll be able to admire your harvest every time you walk into your kitchen!

See, drying and storing herbs isn't so painful after all, is it?

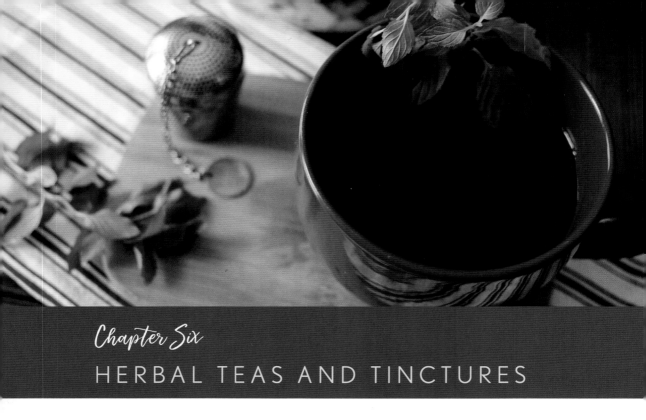

Chapter Six
HERBAL TEAS AND TINCTURES

You've come in from a morning in the garden, and you sit back and admire the harvest you've reaped. The chamomile flowers and stinging nettle you just harvested are absolutely gorgeous. Suddenly you stop and think, *What the heck am I supposed to do with them now?!*

This is the place most people come to in herbalism. They've done all of their research on what these herbs do, but then become overwhelmed with how to use them, what to make with them, and how they work in external and internal herbal preparations. We know how to cook with herbs, which we'll talk about in another chapter, but what about creating health products with them?

The romanticism of creating a product that can essentially help your body, or your animal's health, is rejuvenating. It's exciting. Not only that, but incorporating herbs into your daily life by replacing chemical household products, soaps, cleaners, lotions, medicines, and more with herbal options really brings an entirely new sense of self-sustainability and accomplishment.

All that said, you don't *have* to do it all. The goal is to create a homestead that you're proud of when it comes to the products you use and the food you cook. The key, however, is to not beat yourself up about it if you simply don't have the time to make and cure soap (like me!) or if you just don't enjoy making tinctures (although I encourage you to do it!). You always have a choice. Choose what makes you joyful and leave the rest to people who are passionate about the other creations.

The things that you choose not to make can be bartered through other homesteaders. Or better yet, the things *you make* can be bartered as well.

Homesteaders lean on each other because, let's face it, many of us are parents, farmers, milk maids, nose wipers, egg collectors, garden planters, doctors, and vegetable canners. Adding one more thing to the mix can be overwhelming.

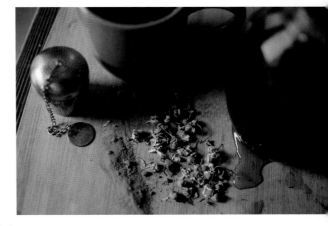

But, *it doesn't have to be.* I think you'll find that much of the practical advice and many of the recipes I'll give you are easy to adapt to your own liking and to your own schedule. You can absolutely be an herbal homesteader—not only growing your herbs but also getting the most out of them.

I'll break down ways to use your herbs one by one, specifically for your health. We'll start with infusions and decoctions, which are basically just fancy terms for teas. These infusions are the things that you can add to your daily diet (so you can eat and drink your medicine!) or consume when you need a health boost. Next, we'll talk extensively about tinctures, as they are the more aggressive line of defense when something is ailing you or your livestock.

HERBAL TEAS AND INFUSIONS

There's nothing better than sitting down to that first cup of herbal tea in the morning. The aroma is most pleasing to the senses, and the taste can be equally as lovely. I'll admit, when I first began drinking herbal teas and infusions, I had to get used to the taste. Let's face it, I'm a Southern mama who loves her sweet iced tea (nowadays, with lemon balm or spearmint!). That's about as close as I got to any type of tea. But as my interest in herbalism grew, I became more and more interested in these extractions.

Herbal teas and infusions are generally your first line of defense when you're in need of a health boost, but they are not necessarily aggressive enough if you're already very sick. Teas are also used to make herbal lotions and soaps. Infusions can be made in tea form to be ingested, or they can even be used in compresses. They are more palatable than some other forms of herbal remedies, and can be made on demand. I should note here that since herbal infusions and decoctions are water-based, they only have a shelf life of about twelve hours.

You don't just have to enjoy herbal infusions when you're sick, however. Herbal teas are a fabulous way to boost your overall health and wellness, and are mainly used for this reason when taken as part of your regular diet. And honestly, they are just downright tasty.

Herbal infusions can also be given to your pets and livestock. In fact, I use them often, like when I place thyme and garlic in my chicken waterers to infuse their drinking water. This ensures that I can boost the entire flock's overall health and support their respiratory systems.

DECOCTIONS AND INFUSIONS: WHAT'S THE DIFFERENCE?

There are two different types of water extractions: **decoctions** and **infusions.**

Decoctions are made with herbs that need to be boiled down. The word "decoction" derives from Latin roots that mean "to boil down." This method is necessary for herbs that don't tend to have volatile essential oils that will be damaged by boiling. The herbs we use in decoctions need to be boiled down in order to release all of their beneficial properties. Most of the time, these herbs are roots, dried berries, seeds, bark, and herbs that are tightly bound together.

Infusions are what we refer to most often when we're creating a tea. Infusions are when you pour boiling, hot, or cold water over herbs and allow them to infuse into the water. These herbs are only allowed to steep for a designated amount of time. We typically only steep these herbs for 5–7 minutes; otherwise, we begin to lose the volatile oils that are in the herbs. If we were to boil these herbs in a decoction, we would lose all of the beneficial essential oils and nutritional components. This is why we make an infusion (or tea), not a decoction, with these types of herbs. We use herbs that have leaves, flowers, and are generally not very dense for infusions.

Here are some of my favorite tea recipes using dried herbs (1 part for me is usually equal to a 1-cup measure):

Making your own tea mixes

You can make your very own tea mixtures at home by mixing various dried herbs into a jar or container and infusing 1–3 teaspoons of the mixture in an 8-ounce cup of hot water as needed. Combine all herbs in a large mason jar, mix well, label, and cap tightly until ready to use. Toss the tea out within 12 hours of steeping it. The entire jar of dried herbs can last from 8–12 months, but will begin to lose its potency after that.

Peppermint Tea

I have a fondness for Hispanic
food and its rice and bean dishes.
Often I have to chase it with
some peppermint tea to help
with digestion, upset stomach,
and bloat. It has also helped me
through several bouts of gluten
intolerance flare-ups.

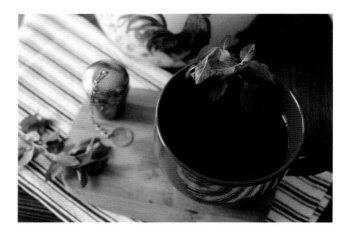

1 part peppermint leaf
½ part lemon balm
¼ part clove, ground

Boost-of-Energy Tea

This tea mixture is perfect for those early mornings when you really just need
a pick-me-up alternative to coffee. Not only do these herbs help heighten the
senses and encourage focus, they taste delicious when you watch the sun rise
before you start your chores!

3 parts green tea
1 part peppermint leaf
½ part clove, ground
½ part ginger root
½ part gingko leaf

Sleep-Encouraging Tea

My favorite herb scent and tea are the same—chamomile. Chamomile naturally promotes calmness and sleep. Combined with these other sleep-enhancing and stress-reducing herbs, this tea is not only good before bed, it's also fabulous after a stressful day. You can add cream to this tea as well, if you like. It adds a layer of richness to the tea.

3 parts chamomile

1 part lemon balm

1 part blackberry leaf

¼ part St. John's wort

⅛ part lavender

A spoonful of honey

Here's a tip! Add 1–2 tablespoons of raw honey to your teas to help cleanse the body and to naturally sweeten your teas. It's also a hit when trying to get your little ones to drink their herbs.

Cough-Relief Tea

The first time I made thyme tea for my son when he had a cough, I thought it might kill the poor fella, knowing how potent thyme can be at times (no pun intended). But surprisingly enough, thyme tea is exceptionally delightful. Combined with these cough-fighting and soothing herbs, this tea is a great cough and sinus reliever for children and adults alike. Add a tablespoon of raw honey to seal the deal with the younger farmhands!

1 part green tea (optional)

1 part thyme

½ part licorice root

¼ part lemon peel

½ part ginger root

Pick-Me-Up Detox Tea

This tea naturally promotes detoxification in the body thanks to the green tea and dandelion root. This is a great tea to start the year off right with weight loss (though it won't make you lose weight), and to naturally rid your body of all those nasties. It's also great when you're feeling sluggish or just need a cleanse. Drink this tea once or twice a day for 4–8 weeks to promote detoxification.

3 parts green tea

1 part peppermint

1 part nettle leaf

1 part dandelion root

½ part cinnamon

¼ part ginseng root

Anti-inflammatory Tea

Turmeric is a staple in our household, whether it's in capsule or tea form. Turmeric tea is one of the greatest teas to have on hand. This tea naturally helps the body reduce inflammation. But watch out, it can get a little spicy from the turmeric and ginger. Add cream to this recipe once it has steeped to create a smoother texture.

2 parts green tea

1 part turmeric

½ part ginger

½ part spearmint (or peppermint)

½ part lemon peel

OTHER WAYS TO MAKE TEAS

As you learn more about herbs, you'll find that the number of tea mixtures is endless. You can start with a base tea, like green, white, or black. Or you can go straight to the herbs. Use the herbs listed in this book to help you create the teas necessary for what your body needs. The more potent herbs should be used in smaller parts than the less potent herbs.

ALL ABOUT HERBAL TINCTURES

Next on the list of ways to use your herbs you'll find tinctures. Alcohol and herbs: That's basically what a tincture is. Sign me up, friend! Just kidding, I'm not that hard-core. Besides, it's a little more in-depth than that. It's also one of my first lines of defense when I want to use an herb to aggressively treat something.

We use tinctures when we know we need a quick remedy to whatever is ailing us. A tincture is an herbal extraction where you extract all of the beneficial compounds of the fresh or dried herb by macerating it in alcohol or glycerin for 2–6 weeks. Typically, it's best to allow the tincture to sit for at *least* four weeks.

Herbal tinctures are one of the most common ways to treat the body when it comes to herbalism. Not only that, but when stored properly—in a colored glass bottle out of heat and sunlight—glycerite tinctures can last from 18–24 months, and alcohol tinctures can last up to six years. With very few herbs and very little effort, you can make an abundance of tinctures that could last you over a decade.

Tinctures are obviously not something that you can make as soon as you need them. You'll want to have them in your medicine cabinet before the need arises. Tinctures can be given to both your human and animal loved ones. Of course, dosing would be different and should always go by weight, based on the herbs. We've given tinctures to even our smallest livestock, like our rabbits (you'll find those tinctures and dosages in the livestock portion of this book).

There are many different ways to make a tincture. The old-fashioned method basically consists of throwing some herbs in a jar, covering them with alcohol, and letting them sit, and then shaking them every day for four weeks. There's the more controlled method, which I prefer, that measures the herbs by weight and the liquid by volume. I can be confident knowing that the dosages are appropriate and that they'll work since I know the exact amount of herb that has been extracted. I can be confident in knowing that what I'm giving my family will not harm them.

Far too often we read recipes for tinctures that are inaccurate. You could just be making an herbal-flavored alcohol with watered-down medicinal properties. Or worse, you could be making a too-highly-extracted tincture that could send your body into dry heaves. (I may have been slightly dramatic on that last part, but I think you get the point.)

The point is, let's get this right the first time, so that we can claim the product works instead of just hoping it does. Let's make sure that if we are going to share that product, or use it on our children, that we know exactly what they are receiving. Therefore, I encourage you to measure out your herbs as much as possible so that you know the exact weight of the amount of herbs that you placed into your tincture, compared to the volume of your alcohol. We'll talk about this more in a moment, but until then, let's get started on making and taking tinctures.

TINCTURE DOSAGE, RATIO, AND SAFETY

Tinctures are incredibly easy to make and even more incredibly efficient. A little bit really does go a long way. Typical doses are 5–30 drops under the tongue 1–3 times a day. However, more intense herbs, like echinacea, may be taken in smaller dosages. It varies based on herb and intensity. Ten to thirty drops may seem like a large range, but I often tell people that the standard dose is a dropperful, or 30 drops.

There are two liquids with which you can make a tincture: alcohol and glycerin.

A 1-ounce bottle dropper typically holds 30 drops of tincture. A dropper from a 2-ounce bottle can sometimes hold 40 drops of tincture, but generally still tends to hold only 30 drops. **To play it safe, never take more than 1 dropperful at a time.** It's important to start with small dosages with tinctures. Start by taking 5 drops three times a day (15 drops total). If you don't feel relief, up the dosage gradually. **The dosage will depend on your ailment, body type, and the herb that you wish to use.**

Alcohol tinctures are much more common and easier to make, because many people readily have the alcohol available, or it may be easier to come by since you can just run to the local liquor store to purchase it. It also often has a longer shelf life than glycerin. However, alcohol may not be an option for you and your family. Maybe you don't want alcohol in your household, or you don't want to give it to your children. In this case, there are glycerites.

Glycerites are lighter, more palatable, glycerin-based tinctures. We've been using glycerin in pharmaceuticals since the mid-1800s. Glycerin naturally occurs in fats and is water soluble. Most of our glycerin is coconut-oil based; otherwise, it can be soy-based, but coconut is preferred as the body breaks down soy differently.

For either menstruum (solvent liquid) that you use, you'll measure with a weight (w) by volume (v) measurement system. Your weight will be the weight of your herbs, and the volume will be the volume of your alcohol or glycerin. Both should be measured beforehand if at all possible.

The formula

Herb tincture recipes are measured by the ratio of the weight of the herbs to the volume of the liquid (w:v).

Ideal tincture strengths should be a 1:5 or 1:10 ratio. The 1:5 ratio is most common and recommended, while the 1:10 ratio is used for more potent herbs. More

Fresh versus dried

Fresh herb tincture ratio: Fresh herbs hold more moisture; therefore, you may need to decrease your alcohol volume to a 1:2 ratio. Unfortunately, this is sometimes extremely hard with certain herbs because they are more or less dense. A 1:5 ratio is still best, but even striving for less than that is better, as fresh herbs release a lot of moisture during the process. You should also always use 100 proof alcohol for fresh herbs. This causes your mixture to not go rancid since more moisture is being released in your fresh herb tincture.

Dried herb tincture ratio: Because dried herbs have hardly any moisture, they ensure a more accurate ratio conversion. Your ratio should be 1:5 for dried herbs since they don't release moisture. Always use an 80 proof or higher vodka, as it extracts the medicinal properties better and guarantees sterility of the tincture from contaminates.

likely than not, go with the 1:5 ratio. We use this ratio with infused oils and other extractions as well.

What in the world does this ratio thing mean? Well, it's simple math, really. The plant material by weight, by the volume of liquid (w:v) is the ratio, allowing you to understand your tincture strength. Your weight is always the herb, and the volume is always the alcohol or glycerin.

For example, if your tincture were to call for 8 ounces of calendula, with a 1:5 ratio, you would need 40 ounces of alcohol because $8 \times 5 = 40$.

Preparing Your Homestead Tincture

Now that we know the science behind making a tincture, let's dive right into making one.

1 pint mason jar (or larger)

2 oz of herbs

10 oz of alcohol or glycerin

STEP 1:

Select your herb, preferably dried, and weigh out 2 ounces for your jar. I prefer to use a digital kitchen scale that measures in pounds, ounces, and grams. You may find that you need more headspace for less dense herbs, like calendula, in which case, simply use a larger jar. ("Headspace" is the space in the jar from the bottom rim, where the lid screws on, all the way to the top of the jar.) The jar measurements of a mason jar aren't used during the tincture-making process; it's simply the most efficient container to make the tincture in, as glass is the preferred container material when making tinctures.

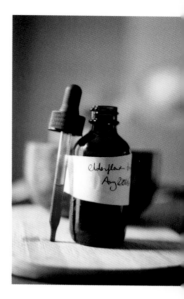

STEP 2:

Push dried herbs down as much as possible to help create more headspace in the jar. Slowly add the 10 ounces of alcohol or glycerin to your jar, stirring the herbs so that they all become saturated and submerged. Wipe the rim and cap off the jar tightly with a spill-proof top (plastic screw-on lids are best). Label your jar with the date you made the tincture and the date it will be ready to use.

STEP 3:

Set your jar on your countertop or in your pantry, away from direct sunlight and extreme temperature changes. A maceration time period of 2–6 weeks is necessary. Each day, shake your jar to mix the tincture and ensure the herb is extracting well. *Do not* open the jar. *Do not* add more liquid if the herb soaks up much of your original menstruum.

STEP 4:

After six weeks, strain the tincture through a clean towel or cheesecloth into a new, and thoroughly cleaned, glass eyedropper bottle, pressing on the herbs to release all of the liquid that you can. You

Some of my favorite tinctures

These tinctures are all made at the 1:5 ratio:

Echinacea and elderberry: lessens the common cold and flu

Astragalus, wild cherry bark, and elderberry: suppresses cough, lessens the common cold and flu

Burdock: aids in liver function, suppresses boils, aids indigestion, is high in minerals

Dandelion: aids in liver function, detoxification, and skin conditions

Garlic: regulates and lowers blood pressure

can sterilize your glass eyedropper bottle first if you like, but it's not necessary. The alcohol itself sterilizes the inside of the jar once it's poured in. Cap the glass bottle with the dropper top and label your bottle with the herb tincture name, the ratio, and the date. You can also label it for what it can be used for, and the proper dosage, especially if a family member needs help when you're not around. Store your tincture in your medicine cabinet or in a place out of sunlight or extreme temperatures. **Shake your tincture before each use.**

MY POSITION ON THE FOLK METHOD

It's common for some folks to recommend the "folk method" for making a tincture. It might be a recipe passed down by generations or something learned from older generations of herbalists, but it usually means that you're not measuring anything by weight, just by "part." This means that instead of measuring out your 1:5 ratio as 1 ounce of herb to 5 ounces of liquid, you'd actually measure just by 1 "part" herb to 5 "parts" liquid, without the efficiency of measuring things out by weight. With the folk method, you're using fractions instead of precise weight measurements.

I'll be straight here. *I don't use the folk method for making herbal tinctures unless the herbs have extremely low weights that are practically unmeasur-*

able on a scale. The courses I've taken in herbalism have been science- and evidence-based. I've learned about real-life clinical studies done by doctors practicing herbalism. Even the great herbalist James Green himself admits that the folk method isn't always reliable.

While these types of tinctures can be effective, and have been used for centuries, there's no way to tell how much of the herb is actually being extracted, and it also leaves a lot of room for error.

You see, the issue here is that some herbs appear to weigh more or as much as others. I could fill up an entire pint jar with calendula and it would only weigh an ounce. I could also fill up a quarter of a pint jar with lavender and that would only weigh an ounce. See the difference?

Using a weight-to-volume ratio allows me to know what, exactly, is in the tincture I'm making, and the exact amount that I should be giving to my family and friends when it comes to medicinal compounds that have been extracted.

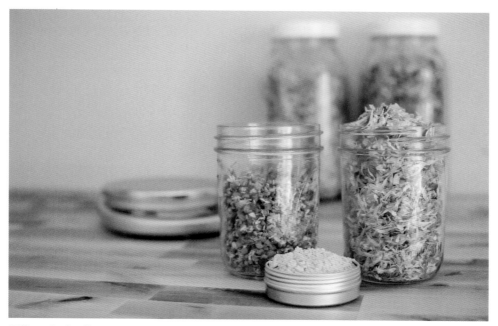

Different herbs all measured out to 1 ounce look completely different in size.

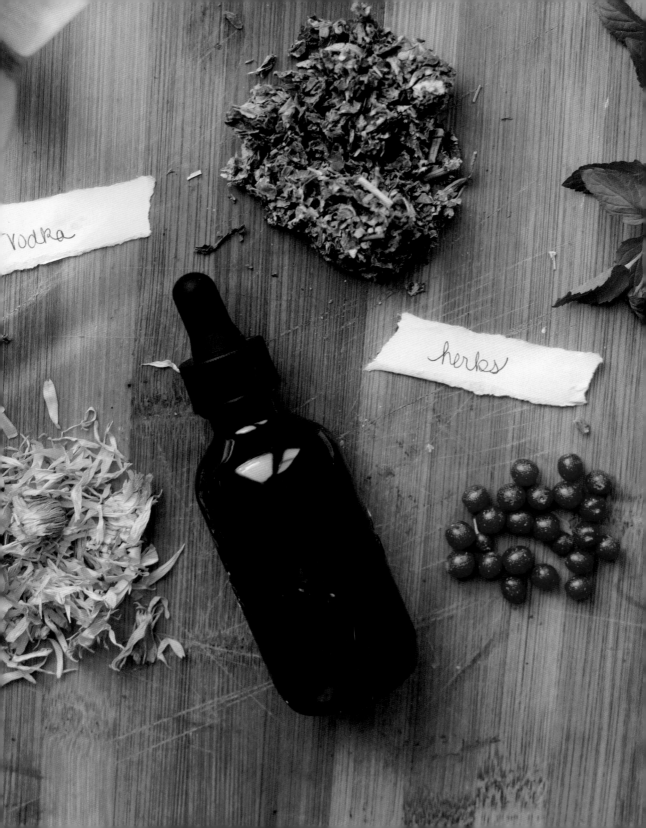

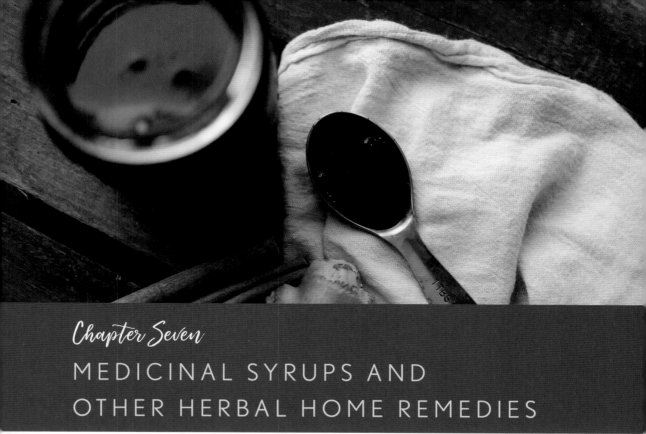

Chapter Seven

MEDICINAL SYRUPS AND OTHER HERBAL HOME REMEDIES

If I had to choose my favorite thing to create with herbs, it would probably be syrups. That's likely because it involves sugar, but oh well, sue me. I like sugar, in its raw evaporated cane juice form, though sugar doesn't always like me. In small amounts, however, sugar absolutely holds its place in herbalism, especially from a scientific standpoint. You see, the sugar in these herbal remedies is what extends their shelf life. *Did you know sugar is a natural preservative?* It absolutely is.

The very first herbal product that I ever created was elderberry syrup for my son when he was sick. After I'd made a few batches, I was hooked. It worked time and time again on his childhood asthma. Even just a small cold could send him into asthmatic attacks, so it was essential for us to find something he could take that wouldn't harm him, and that would help prevent illness or kick it out of his system quickly.

Syrup shelf life

The shelf life of most herbal honeys and syrups is 4–12 months (the more sugar they contain, the longer they last). You can store these syrups in your pantry or in your refrigerator to help extend shelf life even further. Be sure to bottle your syrup in a colored glass bottle (like brown), so that sunlight does not cause it to go bad quickly. Filter your syrup before putting it in the bottle so that no chunks of herbs are floating around, and store it where the temperature doesn't fluctuate. It's best to make these syrups in smaller batches to limit air exposure.

Use the right water

All syrups should be made with distilled or previously boiled water. This takes out all of the impurities that could make your syrup go rancid.

Elderberry syrup was the key for us then, and still is to this day. Even though he no longer has asthma, we still utilize elderberry syrup, and other syrups, to keep us healthy.

Syrups and herbal honeys have been used throughout the centuries. These extracts are easily palatable, sweet, and satisfying, and much easier to take than a tincture, all while having a similarly aggressive approach. We often use herbal blends with honeys and syrups as well.

Syrups and honeys are fabulous for sore throats, as the syrup or honey clings to the inside of the throat when it goes down. Whether it's the change in weather, hay-cutting season, a common cold, or an allergic reaction to an animal, syrups are the way to go.

MAKING A MEDICINAL SYRUP

Syrups can easily be made on demand when you have all of the ingredients, and they will fill your kitchen with sweet aromas. The beauty of making a syrup is that you can play around with the taste and texture. You can use different herbs to make a blend that attacks certain ailments.

Let's go over a simple elderberry syrup recipe. This is a recipe I've been making on my own for years. In this recipe, we take advantage not only of the medicinal properties of elderberry but also astragalus root (immunity boost), ginger root (tummy soother), and clove (antibacterial, anti-inflammatory, with high amounts of antioxidants).

Dosage:

2 teaspoons once a day as a preventative

1–3 tablespoons every 3–4 hours when sick, until symptoms go away

Shelf life:

3–6 months, longer if refrigerated

Basic Elderberry Syrup

Make this recipe in smaller batches if only using for one or two family members. Double or triple the batch if making for larger families.

100 grams dried black elderberries

20 grams dried astragalus root

15 grams dried ginger root (or powder)

8 grams dried clove

1 quart distilled water (or previously boiled water)

½ cup organic sugar (or evaporated cane juice), optional

1 cup raw honey

METHOD:

1. In a large saucepan, add elderberries, astragalus, ginger, clove, and water. Bring mixture to a boil, stirring frequently. Cook down this mixture on medium-high heat, stirring frequently, until the mixture has reduced by half. This can take 20–30 minutes.

2. Remove from heat and strain your liquid into a bowl or glass container. Measure your liquid, which will be about 1^1/$_2$–2 cups, most likely.

3. Place your liquid back into saucepan with your sugar.. Keep in mind that the sugar is optional, but necessary to make an actual syrup. Bring your mixture back to a boil, stirring frequently to ensure proper mixing, and boil for 10 minutes, or until your desired consistency. We enjoy a thick honey-like syrup, but you can make it as thin or as thick as you'd like. Consistency is not key.

4. Once your syrup has cooled a bit, add your raw honey and stir until completely dissolved.

5. Funnel your syrup into glass bottles once it's cooled a bit, and cap tightly. Preserving them in the refrigerator promotes shelf life and ensures less bacterial contamination.

Measuring tips

Depending on the recipe, sometimes you'll see ingredients measured out by ounces or grams. Oftentimes herbalists measure things by grams when they are too lightweight (or they aren't measuring a lot) of an herb. We also measure by grams when we need a more specific and precise measurement. Remember these simple conversions while making and creating recipes.

1 gram = 0.04 ounces	6 grams = 0.21 ounces
2 grams = 0.07 ounces	7 grams = 0.25 ounces
3 grams = 0.11 ounces	8 grams = 0.28 ounces
4 grams = 0.14 ounces	9 grams = 0.32 ounces
5 grams = 0.18 ounces	10 grams = 0.35 ounces

You can use this basic recipe with any amount of herbs and many different sweeteners. You can use honey, brown rice syrup, sugar, or any other natural sweetener that you prefer, or you can combine sweeteners.

Play around with the recipes by adding or taking away herbs. For example, adding wild cherry bark to the mixture will help with coughing that may be brought on with a cold. Adding mullein can help with upper respiratory issues.

Basic Medicinal Syrup

Make a medicinal syrup with any herbs using this basic method:

5–7 ounces of herbs (total weight)

1 quart distilled water

½ cup sugar

1 cup honey

METHOD:

1. Boil herbs and water until reduced by half.

2. Strain herbs from mixture and put mixture back in saucepan on the stove.

3. Add sugar and boil until desired thickness.

4. Allow mixture to cool a bit, then stir in honey until dissolved.

5. Store in a glass eyedropper bottle in the pantry or fridge.

MAKING FLAVORED SYRUPS

Not everything with herbs has to be medicinal. You can make flavored syrups with herbs as well. Many times, they can also be medicinal. Sometimes we just use them to drizzle over ice cream or pancakes, in teas and drinks, and over cheeses. Flavored syrups can be sweet or savory. But all are made basically the same way.

Flavored syrups also work well to mask the unpleasant taste of medicine. For example, making a syrup out of chamomile and mint will hide a tincture flavor very well.

Some of my favorite flavored syrups:

Wild Violet

Chamomile and Wild Violet

Chamomile and Lavender

Peppermint and Thyme

Thyme

Lemon Balm and Peppermint

Ginger and Lemon Balm

Ginger and Clove

Basil, Garlic, and Rosemary

Cayenne, Garlic, and Thyme

Simple Wild Violet Syrup

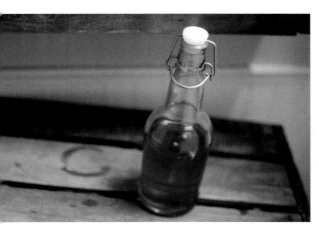

One of my favorite syrups to make in the spring is wild violet syrup. Just about everyone has wild violets growing around them somewhere, and their wild taste goes fabulously in a glass of sweet tea. Have I mentioned lately how much I love sweet tea? Wild violets have more vitamin C than oranges, and more vitamin A than spinach. That's a pretty big deal! They are a lovely wild herb to forage for each spring. We can boil this goodness down into a syrup that gives us a fresh springtime flavor, but is also healthy for the gut and body. Wild violets are one of those things that I simply don't measure out very often. If I were making a medicated syrup to be taken frequently or in large amounts, I would certainly go through the measuring process. But it's not necessary in flavored syrups that are used sparingly.

2 cups boiling water

1 cup violet flower tops, fresh (½–¾ cup if dried)

1½ cups organic sugar (or evaporated cane juice)

1 tsp fresh lemon juice

METHOD:

1. Pick and clean your violet flower tops gently.

2. Place your flower tops in a large bowl or glass and pour 2 cups of boiling water over the violet tops to create an infusion. Your water will turn blue over the next hour or two.

3. After allowing your infusion to sit for 1–2 hours, strain into a clean saucepan, squeezing out as much liquid as you can from the flower tops.

4. Add sugar and bring to a boil. Stir your mixture frequently for about 8–10 minutes or until it reaches your desired consistency.

5. Remove from heat and add lemon juice. If you used regular white sugar, your syrup will turn a violet color. If you used a natural sweetener, like the evaporated cane juice, your liquid will turn a rosy or brownish color.

6. Place your syrup in a glass bottle, cap tightly, and keep in the refrigerator for up to six months.

Basic Flavored Herb Syrup

Make any flavored syrup with any herbs using this basic method:

1–2 cups herbs (fresh or dried)

4 cups distilled water

1½ cups sugar

1 tsp fresh lemon juice (optional)

½ cup fruit, pureed (optional)

METHOD:

1. Boil herbs and water until reduced by half. If using fresh herbs, you can make a simple infusion first, and then do step 2.

2. Strain herbs from mixture and put mixture back in a saucepan on the stove.

3. Add sugar. If using fruit, add pureed fruit to saucepan as well. Boil until desired thickness.

4. Store in a glass bottle in the fridge and use to drizzle over culinary delights like pancakes, cheeses, and more.

USING HONEY AS A DELIVERY SYRUP

We call raw honey "liquid gold" around here. Honeybees are treasured by every single farmer and homesteader. We know the hard work that they go about each and every day. Raw honey is to be praised! Amen.

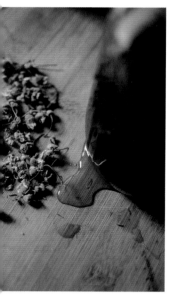

Raw honey has so many incredible medicinal benefits. It heals wounds, it's antibacterial, it counteracts pollen and allergies, has natural antioxidants, and aids as a natural cough syrup. This stuff is amazing, if I do say so myself. Want to hype it up even more? Try manuka honey.

Whenever we refer to an herbal honey, it's basically where we take raw honey and add something to it so it's more palatable, like digestible essential oils, tinctures, glycerites, or powdered herbs. But we can also infuse herbs into raw honey.

This is where we are able to take advantage of the nutritional components of honey and herbs together, rather than losing them during the boiling process. While I always prefer to make syrups with sugar and honey, this is a great alternative when you're in a pinch and you don't have time to make a syrup. Of course, extracted syrups really should be made beforehand anyhow, or when you want to use raw honey as a means to heal the body.

Raw Honey Note: When using raw honey in syrups, you're not using it for its medicinal properties, as those are destroyed during the boiling process. You are using honey as a means to deliver the herbal medicine as a natural sweetener. You can use organic processed honey, but we always have raw honey on hand on our homestead.

You can certainly add the raw honey after the mixture begins to cool to maintain its medicinal properties. However, you'll need to store the syrup in the fridge to ensure a longer shelf life.

Here are great recipes for using honey as a delivery truck with essential oils.

Eucalyptus and Lemon Cough Syrup

I was skeptical when I first heard of making cough syrup with essential oils, but I became a believer when I was at the end of a long night with my little boy who had been coughing his head off. I first saw a similar recipe created by Jessie Hawkins of The Vintage Remedies Learning Center, but we were able to tweak it for our own needs. This cough syrup absolutely works; however, a little really does go a long way!

4 tbsp raw honey

3 drops eucalyptus (*E. radiata*) essential oil

2 drops peppermint essential oil

4 drops lemon essential oil

METHOD:

1. Mix well in a glass jar. Cap tightly when not in use. Keeps for 3–7 days.

2. When needed, administer $^1/_2$ tablespoon by mouth every 4–6 hours (ages 7+ only).

Soothing Ginger Honey Syrup

This syrup is great when your stomach is upset or when you're nauseated. Ginger and peppermint are known to soothe upset stomach and to aid digestion. This is great after a holiday meal or when you've eaten something that doesn't agree with you. It's also great for stomach flu.

4 tbsp raw honey

3 drops ginger essential oil

2 drops peppermint essential oil

METHOD:

1. Mix well in a glass jar. Cap tightly when not in use. Keeps for 3–7 days.

2. When needed, administer 1/2 tbsp by mouth every 4–6 hours.

You can also use honey to administer powdered herbs and supplements. We all remember our mamas putting our vitamins or medicine in applesauce or honey, and that same method works well today. Something so simple, yet so effective!

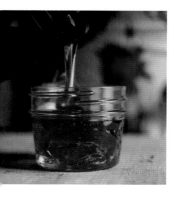

HERB-INFUSED HONEYS

Honeys can also be infused with herbs, much like we infuse herbs in oil. This is mostly done to enjoy the taste of the herbs, not always for the beneficial compounds that are within them. However, they can work both ways. I especially enjoy using infused raw or manuka honey as a healing agent on wounds. Infusing the honey with herbs simply enhances that medicinal quality even more. Here are some of my go-to herbal honey recipes.

Basic Infused Herbal Honey

1 oz dried herbs

5 oz raw local honey

METHOD:

1. Place ingredients in mason jar (making sure the herbs are completely covered with honey), cap tightly, and set in a sunny windowsill or warm area for two weeks. Turn jar over once in the morning and once in the evening to mix ingredients.

2. Once desired aroma and taste is acquired, strain herbs from honey. Place infused honey in new glass jar and cap tightly. Store in pantry.

3. Drizzle over culinary dishes, desserts, or take as a dietary supplement.

All of these infused honeys can be used in culinary dishes, and many can be used for medicinal purposes as well. Raw honey alone has amazing medicinal qualities. Why not eat your medicine?!

Don't worry about your honey going rancid or being contaminated. Honey is a natural antibacterial, and as long as your herbs are completely submerged in honey, there shouldn't be an issue.

Goes great with honey

Garlic	Ginger
Lavender	Rosemary
Thyme (great for coughs)	Basil
Lemon Balm	Lavender
Peppermint	Chamomile

Lavender and Chamomile-Infused Honey

The nutty, apple, and floral tastes that arise from this honey are exhilarating. This is an infused honey that you'll want to keep on hand for the rest of your life. This honey is great for teas and ice cream, but play around with it in baking, and even use it on wounds and bug bites!

1 oz lavender buds, dried

1 oz chamomile flowers, dried

8–10 oz raw honey

METHOD:

1. Add dry herbs to the bottom of a mason jar. You may need to crush up your herbs a bit to ensure the honey covers them.

2. Pour raw honey over herbs and carefully mix.

3. Cap tightly and set on your counter or in a cool dark place for 2–3 weeks.

4. Strain herbs from honey and use the honey on top of sweet breads, ice cream, or in teas and mixed drinks. You can also use this honey directly on wounds, as the honey is naturally antibacterial.

Herbal Healing Infused Honey

It's well known among herbalists and natural remedy users that raw honey has healing properties. Adding herbs to your honey just enhances those healing properties even more. In this recipe I use herbs that are known to soothe and heal, and that are naturally anti-inflammatory. This infusion is a powerhouse for cuts, scrapes, and minor and severe wounds. Simply apply to affected area, cover with gauze or a bandage, and allow to absorb for 8–10 hours before re-dressing.

1 oz chamomile flowers, dried

1 oz plantain, dried

1 oz yarrow, dried

10 oz manuka honey (or raw honey)

METHOD:

1. In a large bowl, crush up dried herbs.

2. Add herbs to a large mason jar, and cover with raw honey.

3. Allow to sit on the counter or in your dark pantry for 2–3 weeks, shaking every day or so.

4. Strain herbs from honey, cap tightly, label, and store for up to one year.

5. External use only (wounds, cuts, burns, etc.).

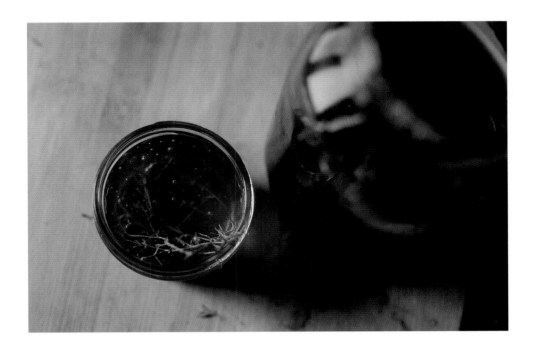

What's the fuss about manuka honey?

Want an even greater result for external-use, infused honeys? Swap out raw honey for manuka honey. Now we're talking, baby! Manuka honey is derived from bees that pollinate manuka bushes in New Zealand. It can be up to four times more powerful in antibacterial properties than regular raw honey. Science itself has even confirmed the many benefits of manuka honey. In 2010, the National Cancer Institute approved clinical trials to test whether the honey might aid in reducing inflammation in the esophagus of patients receiving chemotherapy. Studies have shown it to be powerful in healing even severe wounds and burns, oftentimes helping skin naturally regenerate. Manuka honey is high in amino acids, B vitamins, calcium, magnesium, potassium, and more. We typically only suggest external use for higher therapeutic grade manuka honey.

Here's how to tell what UMF (Unique Manuka Factor) grade you have: http://www.umf .org.nz/grading-system-explained

0–4 nontherapeutic grade

4–9 comparative to raw local honey

10–14 increased bacteria fighting properties.

15+ advanced levels that are highly therapeutic. If using internally, never take more than 1 tablespoon at a time.

If you want the best for external use, go with a 10–15. For internal use that exceeds raw honey's abilities, stick with 10–14. You can find these numbers on most labels of manuka honey. You can purchase this honey online or in specialty food stores.

USING APPLE CIDER VINEGAR

You can also make tinctures and liquid extractions with apple cider vinegar and other acidic liquids, but it is less common. Instead of using vodka, glycerin, or honey for these ingestible extractions, use apple cider vinegar. Raw apple cider vinegar has amazing health benefits, and is probably most notably known for helping the body remain alkaline and balancing out acidity levels in the gut.

The best apple cider vinegar to use is raw apple cider vinegar containing the "mother." The mother is a portion of the bacteria disc that is bottled with the vinegar. This bacteria was used to create the vinegar itself. Choosing this vinegar allows your vinegar to continue to ferment and retain beneficial bacteria for each use.

One of my favorite ways to use apple cider vinegar is to make fire cider. Whew, what a kick-butt extraction this is! Fire cider is typically one of those extractions that I simply don't measure. There is so much heat in this extraction that it's enough to burn the hairs off your nose. But for many people, the special blend of this extraction helps cure whatever ails them. And yes, it really does work.

People like my husband—you know, the big burly type—for some reason just love fire cider. He swears up and down that it works ten times better than elderberry syrup for him. And honestly, for his body type, I do believe he's right. Some people just need a bigger kick in the rear when it comes to herbal medicine. But I believe that it's mainly because fire cider is naturally anti-inflammatory. For people who deal with inflammation frequently, this is the remedy for them.

Fire cider is extremely hot and tangy, but has major health benefits from the herbs contained in it. It is anti-inflammatory, antiviral, antibacterial, helps the circulatory system, and can even act as a decongestant. In other words, when the common cold says, "I'm going to get you, human being," the human being responds, "Hold my beer."

Fire Cider

DOSAGE:

1 teaspoon of cider every 3 hours until symptoms subside. Or 1 shot glass a day to keep the doctor away.

Some people say that taking a shot each day helps to keep cold and flu away, but this has not yet been scientifically proven. However, with the amount of garlic and ginger, and heat, I wouldn't toss that theory to the side! In general, this tonic is a great dietary supplement to take each day to help with inflammation, blood circulation, and overall health.

½ cup fresh ginger root, peeled and roughly cut

¼ cup fresh turmeric, peeled and roughly cut

½ cup fresh horseradish root, peeled and roughly cut

½ cup onion, peeled and diced

¼ cup garlic, peeled and roughly cut

½ cup jalapeno peppers, chopped, seeds in

zest and juice of 2 lemons (measure liquid if possible)

3–4 cups organic raw apple cider vinegar (with the mother)

raw organic honey

METHOD:

1. In a quart-size mason jar, add all dry ingredients, plus lemon zest and juice. You can place a fermenting weight on top of your dry ingredients, or you can leave them be.

2. Add 3–4 cups of raw apple cider vinegar to your quart jar. This will most likely fill your jar almost completely to the top. Leave a 1-inch headspace, as some of your root herbs may expand.

3. Cap the jar tightly with a plastic screw top, shake well, and set the jar in your pantry or in a place out of direct sunlight and extreme temperatures.

4. Allow your tincture to macerate for four weeks, shaking once each day.

5. After four weeks, strain your liquid into a new glass jar and dispose of the herbs. Add up to 1 cup of honey, or more, until you reach the desired taste and consistency. Label with name, ingredients, and date.

Note: This extraction is best kept in the refrigerator for an extended shelf life. General shelf life is up to six months in the refrigerator.

HERBAL CONFECTIONARIES FOR THE MINI HERBALISTS

We all know that a spoonful of sugar helps the medicine go down, but what about involving the mini herbalists into the mix with homemade herbal confectionaries? Not only does it give them a sense of accomplishment that they made their own medicine, it's also just fun to eat your medicine when it's on the other end of a lollipop stick, right?! Make sure younger children aren't around during the sugar-boiling process, as hot sugar can be painful if it shoots out of the pan. Mini farmhands can help weigh everything, and they can help spray the pan down, but otherwise, they make the best bystanders.

Immune-Boosting and Cough-Relieving Lollipops (or Drops)

DOSAGE:

1 lollipop or cough drop every 2–4 hours

2½ cups distilled water

1 oz black elderberries, dried

½ oz wild cherry bark, dried

¾ oz astragalus root, dried

¼ cup cherry or grape juice (or any fruit juice will do)

1 cup evaporated cane juice (or raw sugar)

1 cup honey

METHOD:

1. In a saucepan, combine water and dried herbs. Bring to a boil and decoct at a rolling simmer for 30 minutes. Make sure the water doesn't evaporate or hard boil during that time.

2. Strain the herbs from the liquid. You'll be left with about ½ cup of liquid. Add ¼ cup of cherry or grape juice to the liquid. Return to saucepan.

3. Add honey and cane juice to the saucepan and boil mixture until it reaches 300°F (use a candy thermometer).

4. Quickly remove from heat and pour into coconut-oiled lollipop molds or by drops on a cookie sheet lined with parchment paper.

5. Allow to cool completely and then package individually or in a freezer bag. Label and store for up to three months.

Tummy-Soothing Ginger Chews

DOSAGE:

2 chews every 2–4 hours (adults), 1 chew every 2–4 hours (children)

4 tbsp coconut oil

2 oz fresh ginger, peeled and shredded

½ cup honey

¾ cup evaporated cane juice (or raw sugar)

5–8 drops lemon essential oil

METHOD:

1. In a saucepan, combine coconut oil and fresh ginger. Warm on a low heat setting for 20 minutes, infusing the oil with the herb.

2. Strain out the ginger from the oil. Place oil back in saucepan with honey and evaporated cane juice and bring to a boil.

3. Continue to stir mixture until candy thermometer reaches 245°F–250°F. Remove from heat, but continue stirring until all the bubbles subside. Then add the lemon essential oil.

4. Pour mixture into a prepared baking dish or sheet (lined with parchment paper or greased with coconut oil). Allow to cool for 30–60 minutes.

5. Turn out cooled mixture onto a flat surface covered with confectioner's sugar (optional). Cut chews into bite-size squares and wrap individually. Store in an airtight container for 6–8 weeks.

Herbal Gummies

These gummies are really fun for the little ones to help you make. Make elderberry gummies for cold and flu season, or make other gummies by switching out the herbs!

¼ cup grape concentrate

½ cup hot water

⅓ cup gelatin

1 cup homemade elderberry syrup (see recipe on page 127)

Gummy molds

METHOD:

1. In a large bowl, quickly whisk together grape juice concentrate, hot water, and gelatin.

2. Add in elderberry syrup and stir quickly.

3. Pour mixture into coconut-oiled gummy molds. Refrigerate for 1 hour, then pop out into a gallon bag and keep in the fridge for 1–2 weeks.

Note: If you don't want to use immune-boosting elderberry syrup, try using vegetable juices, infusions, and decoctions! If you don't have a concentrate on hand, just use juice. Concentrates are the liquid left over after water has been removed from a juice.

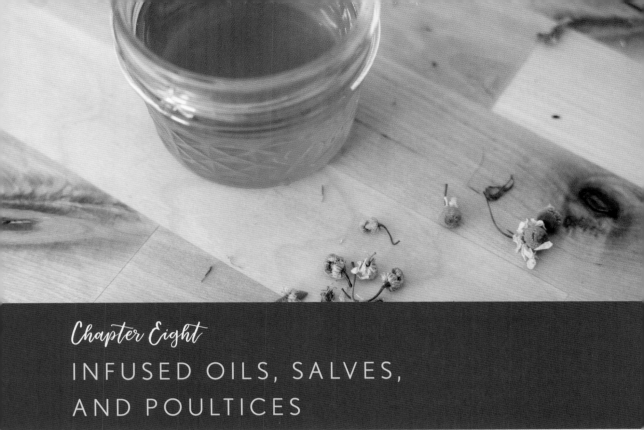

Chapter Eight

INFUSED OILS, SALVES, AND POULTICES

The basis for so many other herbal products, like lotions, salves, and balms, begins with herb-infused oils. Herb-infused oils are also great for massage therapy, or when you simply need a quick, absorbing topical remedy.

You can make infused oils two different ways. The first way is much like making a tincture, except you're using an oil rather than vodka, to extract the beneficial compounds of the herb during a 2-4 week process. The second way is the way I prefer because I don't often keep infused oils on hand. In the second method, you simply add your herb to your oil and heat it in the oven at a low temperature for 2-4 hours. If you don't want to put it in the oven, you can heat it on a very low heat over a double boiler for 2-3 hours.

This is the most common method in the Fewell household because, let's face it, I'm a mom and when I need to make a salve, I don't want to have to wait 2-4 weeks before I can use it.

Infused Oils the Slow Way

½ oz of herbs

1–1½ cups of oil (fractionated coconut oil, olive oil, or grapeseed oil)

METHOD:

1. Combine all ingredients in a glass mason jar. Cap tightly and allow to sit in a sunny area for 2–4 weeks, shaking occasionally each day.

2. Once infused, strain out herbs, capturing all of the infused oil in a new glass. Cap tightly and store in your cabinet for up to six months.

Infused Oils the Quick Way

½ oz of herbs

1–1½ cups of oil (coconut, olive, or grapeseed oil)

METHOD:

1. Preheat oven to 300°F.

2. Combine herbs and oil in an ovenproof dish so that herbs are completely covered with oil. Add dish to preheated oven, turn oven off and allow the mixture to infuse in the oven heat for 2–3 hours.

3. Strain out herbs from the infused oil while still warm. Place oil in a glass bottle, cap tightly, and store in your cabinet for up to six months.

You can also use a double boiler or put jars in your crockpot to make your infused oils. All methods typically use the same amount of herbs and oil (you can double or triple a recipe), but use different heating and extracting methods. The goal is not to cook the herb, but to add just enough heat to begin extracting the beneficial compounds into the oil.

You can use infused oils for all types of things, as mentioned previously. Here are some of my favorite herbs to make infusions with. You can also use all of these infused oils to create salves and other products, or apply them straight from the jar onto your skin.

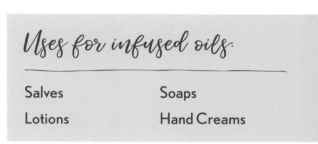

Arnica: For sore muscles, aches and pains, and closed wounds.

Cayenne: For bone and muscle aches, back pain, and occasional soreness.

Chamomile: For soothing irritated skin.

Comfrey: Also known as "knitbone," this oil is great to rub on parts of the body that have broken or fractured bones. It also works well on athlete's foot, and for the regeneration of tissue for conditions like eczema.

Uses for infused oils.

Salves   Soaps

Lotions   Hand Creams

Feverfew: Great for headaches and general health.

Lemon Balm: For wounds and skin conditions, as a mood lifter, or to help calm the central nervous system.

Thyme: Rub on chest to help sooth coughing, use for minor skin irritations and muscle soreness.

Yarrow: Is naturally anti-inflammatory for sore muscles and inflammation on parts of the body, good for muscle spasms.

HERBAL SALVES

Boo-boos, broken bones, and bug bites are inevitable on any farm and homestead. Toss in a little bit of a headache, achy muscles, and hay fever, and you've got what we call there a "farmer." That's right, it happens to the best of us. Straw in our jeans, mud on our boots, and cuts that are bound up with electrical tape or twine because we don't carry Band-Aids

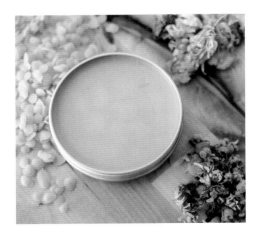

with us when we're mending fences or chasing cows through the neighbor's yard.

Most of the issues you have on a farm will involve some type of cut or wound that needs healing. But the mere fact that we work with our hands on a regular basis should be enough to convince us to keep salves in our medicine cabinet at all times—whether it's for our livestock or for ourselves.

Salves are *so* easy to make and keep on hand. You can make a salve for just about anything—whether it's for a headache, burns and wounds, a knockoff VapoRub, or something for that farm kid's persistent diaper rash.

Makeshift double boiler

When making salves, you'll need to make a double boiler on your stovetop to melt the beeswax and combine everything. Do this by using a saucepan with about 1 inch of water in the bottom. Put on medium heat. Add a mason jar to the saucepan and do all of your mixing in the mason jar.

As you may recall, your salves will begin with infused oils. Don't worry, if you don't have infused oils on hand, you can make them within 2–3 hours. Just refer to the infused oils section of this chapter. Salves are another one of those fabulous herbal products that you can make ahead and keep on hand for later use. They also fit great into farm first aid kits, in the work truck, your pocket, or your purse.

All of these salves can be used not only on you and your family, but on your livestock as well. In fact, the "Black Drawing Salve" recipe in this section is used more often on my livestock than on my family. It's my go-to for frostbitten rooster combs, open wounds, and broken skin.

Herbal salves and balms are a fantastic way to heal, calm, and relieve the body. They can be used to treat a specific issue, or just as a stress reliever. The possibilities are endless with herbal ointments and salves.

Basic Salve Recipe

3–3.5 oz herb-infused oil

.5 oz beeswax

20 drops essential oil (optional)

METHOD:

Melt together in a double boiler, pour into tins, allow to cool before capping. Store up to one year.

Simple Soothing Salve

I have this salve on hand at all times. I use it for bumps, bruises, minor skin cuts and scrapes, and more. It soothes the skin, reduces pain, and helps with inflammation. It's our go-to salve!

1 oz calendula-infused oil

1 oz chamomile-infused oil

1 oz arnica-infused oil

.5 to 1 oz beeswax

METHOD:

1. In a double boiler, combine all ingredients until completely melted.

2. Quickly pour into tins and allow to cool completely.

3. Cap tightly, label, and store for up to one year.

Black Drawing Salve

I use this drawing salve mostly on my animals. It works perfectly for frostbitten rooster combs, wounds on legs, and more. Seriously, I put this junk on everything! For anything that needs a thick layer of protection and sealant, and to draw out any infection, this is the salve to use.

6 tbsp calendula-infused oil

3 tbsp plantain-infused oil

1 tbsp coconut oil
(or sweet almond, castor,
or grapeseed oil)

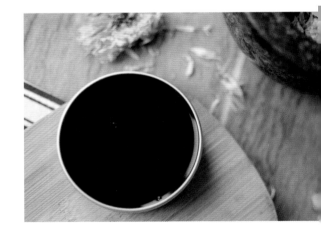

3 tsp beeswax

3 tsp activated charcoal

3 tsp bentonite clay

10 drops tea tree essential oil

10 drops lavender essential oil
(optional)

Storage tins or jars

METHOD:

1. In a saucepan, add about 1 inch of water to the bottom and turn on to medium heat. You're making a double boiler so that your oils won't be touching direct heat.

2. In a glass or tin jar, add calendula oil, plantain oil, coconut oil, and beeswax. Place jar in saucepan to create a double boiler. Stir oils and beeswax until melted completely.

3. Add charcoal and clay; mix well. If you need a thicker consistency, add a little more clay.

4. Remove from heat and add essential oils. I like to add tea tree and lavender because of their healing properties, but the possibilities are endless.

5. *Optional—if you'd like a more whipped consistency, leave the salve in the mason jar until almost hardened, then whip it with a whisk or immersion blender.

6. Pour salve into a jar or individual tins. Allow to cool completely, then cap tightly, label, and store for up to a year in your medicine cabinet.

7. When needed, use a small amount topically. Cover with a bandage for up to 12 hours before rinsing off.

Note: Activated charcoal and bentonite clay can be purchased from most health food stores and online. They can sometimes be found in the health and beauty section of regular stores as well.

Burn and Wound Healing Salve

1.5 oz echinacea-infused oil

1.5 oz plantain-infused oil

.5 oz beeswax

10 drops tea tree essential oil

1 tbsp raw honey (optional)

METHOD:

1. In a double boiler, add infused oils and beeswax, and stir until completely melted and combined.

2. Remove from heat and quickly add essential oil and raw honey (if using).

3. Pour into tins, allow to cool, cap tightly, label, and store in your medicine cabinet for up to one year.

4. Use on burns and wounds to speed up healing and soothe the pain.

Pain-Relieving Salve

¼ cup coconut oil

⅕ oz cayenne (capsicum) powder

1½ tsp beeswax

15 drops peppermint essential oil

4 drops clove essential oil

4 drops helichrysum essential oil

METHOD:

1. In a saucepan, create a double boiler with a mason jar.

2. Add coconut oil, cayenne powder, and beeswax to the mason jar. Stir until completely melted and combined.

3. Remove from heat and add peppermint, clove, and helichrysum essential oils. Mix well.

4. Immediately pour into salve tins. Allow to cool, then cap tightly, label, and store in your medicine cabinet. Use within one year.

5. When ready to be used, rub deeply into sore muscles or external areas where you're having pain. This works great on back and muscle pain, especially.

Warning: Do not use if you're pregnant. If skin irritation appears, discontinue use. Some people are more sensitive to capsicum than others. Never apply to an open wound.

Psoriasis and Eczema Ointment

Notice that this ointment doesn't call for beeswax or infused oils like most of our salves do. In this recipe, we're using the natural healing properties and thick consistency of coconut oil to help create our ointment. You can play around with the consistency of this product for immediate results. Oregon grape root has been known to completely heal the skin of people with psoriasis. However, psoriasis is normally an autoimmune or leaky gut issue. I encourage you to dig deeper if this is something you deal with.

1 cup organic coconut oil

4½ tbsp Oregon grape root, powdered

10 drops lavender essential oil

10 drops frankincense essential oil (optional)

METHOD:

1. In a large jar, combine all ingredients and mix well. If the coconut oil is too hard, soften it up a bit in a double boiler and then add the remaining ingredients.

2. Pour into storage tins, cap tightly, label, and store in your medicine cabinet for up to a year. Use as needed.

Peppermint and Feverfew Headache Salve

When needed, apply this salve to the back of your neck, shoulders, and even on your head when you have a headache or feel a headache coming on.

2 oz peppermint-infused oil

1.5 oz feverfew-infused oil

.5 oz beeswax

10 drops peppermint essential oil

10 drops lavender essential oil (optional)

METHOD:

1. In a double boiler, combine peppermint-infused oil, feverfew-infused oil, and beeswax. Melt until combined.

2. Remove from heat and add essential oils. Immediately pour into storage tins or jars.

3. Allow to cool, cap tightly, label, and store in your medicine cabinet for up to one year.

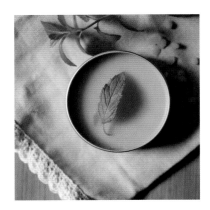

Respiratory Salve

Use as needed, just as you would an over-the-counter mentholated topical ointment during sickness or when in need of respiratory relief. A little goes a long way!

6 tbsp coconut oil

2½ tbsp cocoa butter

2 tbsp beeswax

10 drops peppermint essential oil

10 drops eucalyptus essential oil

5 drops basil essential oil

5 drops tea tree essential oil

5 drops rosemary essential oil

5 drops lemon essential oil

METHOD:

1. In a double boiler, melt coconut oil, cocoa butter, and beeswax. Combine well.

2. Remove from heat and immediately add essential oils, mixing vigorously.

3. Place in containers or tins and allow to cool. Cap tightly, label, and store in medicine cabinet for up to one year.

Bug Bite Salve

This is a very effective and soothing salve for bug bites.

1 oz plantain-infused oil

1 oz chamomile-infused oil

.5 oz beeswax

10 drops lavender essential oil

METHOD:

1. In a double boiler, combine infused oils and beeswax until melted and completely combined.

2. Remove from heat and immediately add essential oil.

3. Quickly transfer salve to containers or lip balm sticks for quick and easy access.

Broken Bone and Sprain Salve

Apply this salve to the affected area multiple times throughout the day to speed up the healing process, lessen bruising, and help ease pain.

2 oz comfrey-infused oil

1 oz St. John's wort–infused oil

.5 oz beeswax

10 drops peppermint essential oil (optional)

METHOD:

1. In a double boiler, combine infused oils and beeswax. Melt and combine thoroughly.

2. Remove from heat and immediately mix in essential oil (if using).

3. Pour into tins, allow to cool, cap tightly, and label. Store for up to one year.

Diaper Rash Salve

Let me explain how this diaper rash salve works. I'm not saying it will be your end-all in every situation, but at first sight of the rash, it should help cure it. The calendula oil helps soothe and regenerate skin cells, the vitamin E oil helps moisturize and allows the healing properties of this oil to soak into the skin, lavender essential oil helps kill the bacteria and yeast, and chamomile essential oil helps soothe the skin. The zinc oxide and beeswax hold it all in!

A little will go a long way, but use as much or as little as you like. Just make sure you apply it to your baby's bottom only and no other sensitive areas.

Skincare superstars

You'll often see calendula and chamomile in salves and skin products as they are the two most effective herbs for skin care.

1 oz calendula-infused oil

1 oz plantain-infused oil

.5 oz vitamin E oil

.5 oz beeswax

.5 oz zinc oxide (optional)

10 drops lavender essential oil

10 drops chamomile essential oil

METHOD:

1. Combine infused oils, vitamin E oil, and beeswax in a double boiler. Mix until melted and completely combined.

2. Turn heat off, but leave jar in double boiler. Add zinc oxide and stir quickly until combined.

3. Remove from heat and immediately add essential oils.

4. Quickly pour salve into tins or jars, allow to cool, cap tightly, label, and store for up to one year.

Calming Salve

Use this salve for those stressful times at work, when your muscles are tense, in times of anxiety, or right before bed when you just need to feel calm and turn your brain off. You'll want to keep this salve with you all the time. It's earthy and delightful, and the calm that it brings is incomparable.

2 oz chamomile-infused oil

10 drops ylang ylang essential oil

5 drops Hawaiian sandalwood essential oil

5 drops vetiver essential oil

5 drops bergamot essential oil

.5 oz beeswax

METHOD:

1. In a double boiler, combine infused oil and beeswax. Stir until completely combined.

2. Turn off the heat and keep the double boiler on the burner. Add the essential oils to the mixture. Remove from heat.

3. Immediately pour salve into tins. Allow to cool completely. Cap tightly, label, and store for up to one year.

Herbal Antibacterial Ointment

I am in love with this natural antibacterial salve. Oregano and raw honey both have antibacterial properties and are incredible at healing the body naturally. I've healed many human and animal wounds with these ingredients, and when they come together in one salve, they are a powerhouse. Use this salve just as you would any over-the-counter antibiotic ointment or salve.

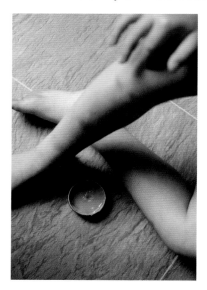

3 oz calendula-infused oil

.5 oz beeswax

10 drops tea tree essential oil

10 drops oregano essential oil

10 drops vitamin E oil

1 tbsp manuka honey

METHOD:

1. In a double boiler, melt together the calendula-infused oil and beeswax.

2. Turn heat off and add essential oils, vitamin E oil, and raw honey.

3. Quickly pour your salve into tins or a jar. Allow to cool completely, then cap, label, and store for up to one year. You can whip the ointment with a whisk or immersion blender if you'd like, but it's not a hard salve so it works well either way.

HERBAL POULTICES

When Junior got pink eye for the third time in a row one year, I couldn't help but wonder if he was just a super active farm kid or if we were living in some type of unclean environment.

Labels for your herb products

Labeling your salves and other herbal products can be such a fun way to express

your creativity. Use graphics on printed labels to brand yourself or your product. You can create these in just about any word processing program. If you're feeling like a more natural look, tie handstamped brown labels with twine to your products, showing the ingredients, uses, and dosage on one side, and your name or a design on the other. Or you can even just write on your tins and bottles with a gold or 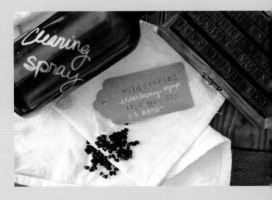 silver permanent marker in a fancy script. I do this most often for the products I make and use at home.

As any modern crunchy mother would do, I reached out to the "interwebs" to see what I could find as a natural alternative. He had already had two rounds of antibiotic eye drops, and I wasn't going that route again.

Next thing I know, I'm reading about this thing called a poultice. *Oh, hello poultice. Nice to finally meet you.* If we're being honest, I wasn't quite sure whether to laugh because it sounded so much like poultry, which is probably where he contracted the pink eye in the first place, or to dive in headfirst to this new herbal discovery.

So, I did both.

I ended up making a garlic poultice, but instead of placing the garlic directly on Junior's eye, I wrapped the garlic pulp in the muslin and placed the little package on or near his eye for thirty minutes every two hours until the symptoms subsided

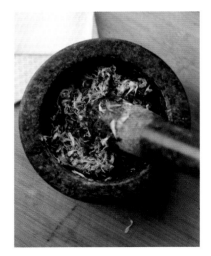

(about one week). Of course, there are different types of pink eye that need different types of treatment (viral versus bacterial), but I was pleased to see this new herbal remedy work for my son.

Herbal poultices are probably one of the most unsung ways to use herbs, simply because most people have no idea what they are, and yet they really aren't intimidating or even hard to create.

So what is a poultice? A poultice is simply another way to apply herbs directly to the skin or to an external part of the body. You accomplish this by grinding the herb into a paste with a mortar and pestle (or food processor). You then apply the herb paste directly to the area that's affected (up to 1 inch thick), wrap it with a bandage so it holds the herb in place, and allow it to set and heal the affected area. A warm or cold poultice can be applied—warm to stimulate circulation, cold to help soothe.

This is a common practice when it comes to older methods of herbalism. Native Americans used poultices, and people who wildcraft— folks who harvest wild plants to make products to use or sell—continue to do so. It's something that I was already doing with plantain leaves from my own backyard whenever we got a bee sting or a cut while out working.

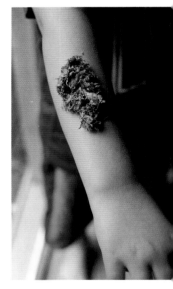

MAKING A FRESH HERB POULTICE

You can make a poultice with fresh or dried herbs, but the methods are a little different. Once you've chosen your fresh herb(s), use enough to make a thick paste with a mortar and pestle. The amount of herbs used will depend on the area you need to cover. There's no need to add liquid—the natural mois- ture in the herbs will create a paste with the herb.

Next, cover the affected area with the herb paste. Then, cover and secure it tightly with a wrap or piece of muslin. Leave the paste on for several hours; it's easiest to use while sleeping. Re-dress and apply as needed.

MAKING A DRIED HERB POULTICE

After choosing your dried herbs, add them to the mortar with a small bit of warm water to begin rehydrating them. If you're using root herbs, it's better to use finely shredded or powdered versions.

Once you reach the desired consistency, apply herbs directly to your skin and cover tightly with a wrap or muslin. Leave on for several hours and re-dress as needed.

Use with caution

If you are pregnant or nursing, please keep in mind that herbs in a poultice will go into your bloodstream. Use with caution and refrain from using herbs that you shouldn't use when pregnant or nursing.

WHEN TO USE POULTICES

Use poultices on wounds, burns, and scrapes. Use them on the chest to help decongest and open airways. You can also use them on areas like the face, but be sure not to apply the herb directly to the skin or any sensitive areas. It's best to wrap poultices in thin pieces of muslin and apply them that way. The natural moisture will soak through the muslin and begin the healing process. Choose from the herb lists in chapters 2 and 4 for the proper poultice based on what needs healing.

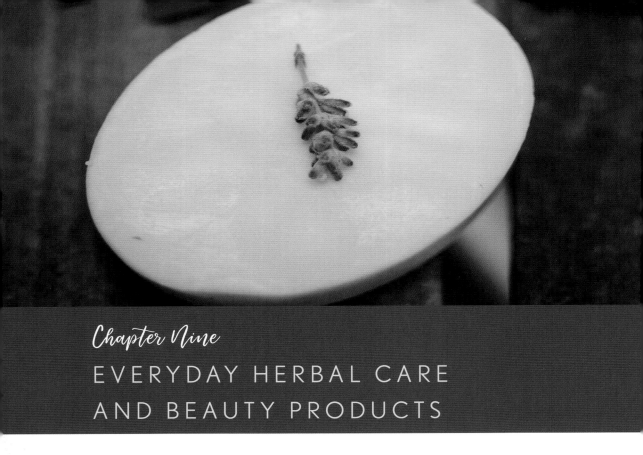

Chapter Nine

EVERYDAY HERBAL CARE AND BEAUTY PRODUCTS

I never realized how many chemicals I used to put on my body on a regular basis, from my face serum and shampoo, to my shaving cream and lip balm. Did you know that some lip balms have petrolatum in them? Do you know what that is? It's a by-product of petroleum. Yuck!

There are many things that we can make easily right in our own homes, with our own herbs and herbal products.

Your skin will definitely appreciate it. It is the greatest organ your body has, and everything that you put onto it seeps deep into your body and bloodstream. If you're constantly using chemical-laden products, you'll end up feeling sluggish, your immune system will suffer, and your body may even begin to react adversely as it tries to rid itself of toxins. When things are going wrong inside the body, oftentimes your skin will tell you.

When you switch to herbal and natural-based products, your body will begin to act differently and actually start to heal itself. When you choose a more natural option and love your body more, you may just find that your body will love you right back.

Here are some options for you as you begin to live a more natural lifestyle.

HERBAL LOTIONS

I have a confession: I don't make lotions very often. I just don't have a great need for lotion. Each year I make one lotion and one farmer's hand cream, and I'm good to go!

Most lotions are made the same way, but you can switch up the infused oils and essential oils for whatever your needs may be. Lotions are a fabulous way to treat the body holistically, but they are mostly used to heal the skin when it's dried out or damaged. Here is a basic lotion recipe, and some other hand and body creams, that any home-steader can make and enjoy!

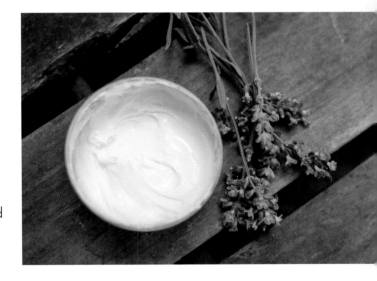

Basic Lotion Recipe

When I reached out to my friend Quinn Veon over at Reformation Acres for my son's chapped skin, she sent us some of her very own homemade lotion. She was even kind enough to give me the Basic Lotion Recipe so that we can make it too!

.5 oz beeswax (pastilles work best)

4 oz moisturizing liquid oil (such as grapeseed, sweet almond, or olive oil)

4 oz water, herbal tea, or hydrosol

10 drops vitamin E

15 drops essential oil of choice (optional)

METHOD:

1. Weigh the beeswax and oil of choice in a wide-mouth mason jar.

2. Place the jar in a small saucepan that has been filled with a couple inches of water. Bring the water to a boil and melt the beeswax in the oil.

3. Remove the jar from the pan and allow it to cool to room temperature. The wax will begin hardening, making the oil cloudy-looking. If you waited too long, just melt it down again.

4. Stir the water, vitamin E, and essential oil together in a separate container.

5. Slowly add the water mix to the oil/beeswax mix while using an immersion blender to whip it to a thick and creamy consistency.

6. Store in a closed container at room temperature for about two months (longer if refrigerated).

Simple Lavender Lotion

Lavender is such a soothing herb. This simple lotion is perfect as an everyday moisturizer, or as a nighttime lotion that promotes restful sleep. With chamomile and lavender together, this lotion proves time and time again to be a favorite in our home. It's also perfect as a gift to a brand new mother, as it's beneficial to mom and baby!

.5 oz beeswax (pastilles work best)

4 oz lavender-infused sweet almond oil

4 oz rose water

10 drops vitamin E

5 drops lavender essential oil

5 drops chamomile essential oil

METHOD:

1. In a double boiler, melt beeswax and lavender-infused almond oil in a wide-mouth mason jar.

2. Remove the jar from the pan and allow it to cool to room temperature until the wax begins to harden.

3. In a separate container, stir together rose water, vitamin E, and essential oils.

4. Slowly add the rose water mix into the oil/beeswax while using an immersion blender to whip it to a thick and creamy consistency.

5. Store in tins or a jar, cap tightly, label, and store for about two months (longer if refrigerated).

Farmer's Hand Cream

This hand cream is fabulous for any farmer, and it's my all-time favorite. When you've been in the garden all day, your hands need extra special attention when the evening comes. Lather up before bed for a soothing scent the entire night, or use this hand cream as needed throughout the day. It is a little greasy, but helps keep all of that moisture in so it renews and revives those skin cells. The calendula and chamomile in this recipe help soothe and regenerate the skin, the essential oils help with inflammation and skin health, as well as skin regeneration, and the butters and beeswax help seal all of that goodness in while doing a mighty fine job at moisturizing as well. Swap out essential oils and infused oils with any other oil options to make hand creams of your own for any type of need!

1 oz cocoa butter

1.5 oz shea butter

1 oz calendula-infused oil

1 oz chamomile-infused oil

.75 oz beeswax

10 drops peppermint essential oil

8 drops helichrysum essential oil

5 drops lavender essential oil

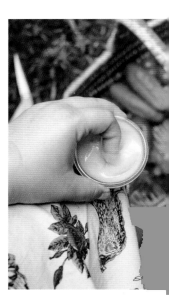

METHOD:

1. In a double boiler, melt down cocoa butter, shea butter, infused oils, and beeswax.

2. Remove from heat and add essential oils.

3. Allow to rest in the mason jar at room temperature (or in the refrigerator) until almost completely hardened. Once it's almost hardened, whip with a whisk or immersion blender.

4. Scoop into a glass jar or into individual tins. Allow to cool completely.

5. Cap tightly, label, and store for up to one year.

Renewing Face Serum

My best friend, Ann Accetta-Scott, made this recipe for her own personal use and now I'm sharing it with you! This lady is into the best years of her life, and she doesn't look a day older than thirty (even though she's in her forties). So when I said, "Give me some of that!" she happily shared her recipe for this the fountain of youth! Because, you know, she's awesome like that. Homestead mamas unite!

I'm going to give you two different versions of this oil to play with—one is Ann's essential oil–based version and the other is a lighter version that also incorporates infused oils that I've put together for you.

Face Serum with Essential Oils

25 drops of frankincense essential oil

25 drops of lavender essential oil

15–20 drops of myrrh essential oil

15–20 drops of geranium essential oil (if you do not like the smell of this oil, keep drops to 15)

carrier oil (fractionated coconut, almond, jojoba, or argan)

METHOD:

1. Fill a 4-ounce eyedropper bottle with the carrier oil of your choice.

2. Add all essential oils, cap, and shake well.

3. Apply 5–10 drops of face serum after you have washed and/or exfoliated your face, typically in the mornings or evenings after a shower. Use within six months.

Face Serum with Essential Oils and Herbs

If you have sensitive skin, reduce the drops of essential oils to half of the amount suggested. This face serum will not only help rejuvenate your skin, it will also help cleanse the skin of any acne-causing bacteria, soothe the skin, and bring radiance to your face.

1.5 oz lavender-infused sweet almond oil

1 oz chamomile-infused sweet almond oil

25 drops of frankincense essential oil

15 drops of myrrh essential oil

10 drops of geranium essential oil

5 drops tea tree essential oil

METHOD:

1. Fill a 4-ounce eyedropper bottle with infused oils.

2. Add all essential oils, cap, and shake well.

3. Apply 5–10 drops of face serum after you have washed and/or exfoliated your face, typically in the mornings or evenings after a shower. Use within six months.

Homemade Powder Foundation Makeup

My skin has been healthier since I ditched the makeup, but sometimes a girl likes to indulge! There's no need to go back to the chemicals, though. Try this all-natural foundation makeup.

¼ cup arrowroot powder

¼ cup kaolin clay

cocoa powder or ground nutmeg (or a mix of the two!)

METHOD:

1. In a jar, combine arrowroot powder and kaolin clay together.

2. Add your cocoa powder or nutmeg ¼ teaspoon at a time until you reach the desired tone for your skin. A little goes a very long way, so don't overdo it on the color!

Note: Store in a jar in your makeup bag and apply as you would any other powder foundation. The nutmeg and cocoa powder really make you smell quite delicious as well. Rock it, girl!

Beard Oil

Many farmers and homesteaders have beards, in case you hadn't noticed. It's a natural source of heat in the winter, and also repels water in the rain and snow. Also, it's just manly. C'mon, let's face the facts. That mane on your face needs just as much attention as the hair on your head. Beard oil is a great product that can be made in just three minutes. Not only does it nourish and condition the facial hair, but also the skin beneath it. The best part about this recipe? You can mix and match any essential oils you want. For a more uplifting serum, try lemongrass and Hawaiian sandalwood. You can even use this serum to provide respiratory relief by using peppermint and eucalyptus. The sky's the limit!

10 drops cedarwood essential oil

3 drops tea tree essential oil

5 drops vetiver essential oil

5 drops white fir essential oil

carrier oil such as jojoba or avocado

METHOD:

1. In a 1-ounce eyedropper bottle, add essential oils.

2. Fill the remaining portion of the bottle up with your carrier oil. If making a larger portion, simply double the oils. Shake well until combined.

3. Apply one eyedropperful to your beard as necessary.

Hair Pomade

This hair pomade is perfect for the fellas who like to look semi-presentable off the farm. Adjust the beeswax in the recipe for a stiffer or softer hold.

1 oz beeswax

1.2 oz shea butter

2 oz jojoba oil (or argan oil)

10 drops tea tree essential oil

10 drops lemongrass essential oil

10 drops rosemary essential oil

METHOD:

1. In a double boiler, combine beeswax, shea butter, and jojoba oil until completely melted and mixed well.

2. Turn heat off and add essential oils.

3. With an immersion blender, begin to blend the mixture until it becomes slightly puffy and light, almost like it's whipped.

4. Transfer your mixture to a container, cap, label, and store for 6–12 months.

Note: Use a very small amount in your hair as needed, adding more as necessary.

Lice be gone!

Want to keep hair pests, like lice, away when you send the kids to school? Add rosemary, eucalyptus, and marjoram essential oils to the pomade hair recipe.

For a stronger hold, add an additional $^1/_2$-1 ounce of beeswax, $^1/_2$ ounce at a time. You can also add vitamin E to this mixture (just a few drops) to help moisturize your hair.

Herbal Lip Balm

The lemon balm in this recipe helps heal the skin of the lips and adds that extra hint of scent and flavor to the mix. Switch up the essential oils for more scents and soothing relief.

1 oz coconut oil

.5 oz lemon balm- or peppermint-infused oil

.5 oz beeswax

.5 oz cocoa butter

20 drops peppermint essential oil

4 drops eucalyptus essential oil (optional)

METHOD:

1. In a double boiler, mix coconut oil, lemon balm–infused oil, beeswax, and cocoa butter. Melt and combine well.

2. Turn heat off and mix in essential oils.

3. Pour mixture into lip balm tubes or individual tins. Allow to cool, then cap tightly, label, and store for up to one year.

Herbal Bath Salts

You can also make this recipe without the herbs and use essential oils instead, such as 7 drops of lavender oil and 7 drops of chamomile oil.

½ cup calendula flowers, dried

1 tbsp crushed rose buds, dried

2 tbsp lavender flower buds, dried

½ cup chamomile flowers, dried

1 cup sweet almond oil or fractionated coconut oil

1 cup sea salt, coarsely ground

1 cup epsom salt

METHOD:

1. In a large bowl, combine all dry ingredients.

2. Add oil and salts into mixture; combine well.

3. Store in a glass container with cap for up to six months.

4. Add 3–4 tablespoons to your warm bath before soaking to promote calmness and muscle relaxation.

HOMEMADE HERBAL DEODORANT

Let's talk about deodorant for a moment, shall we? I'd rather you hear it from me, because I'm going to tell you the brutal and honest truth. And the brutal, honest truth is . . . the first 3–5 days after switching deodorants, you're going to stink!

Your body will go through a detox and pore-cleansing period, especially if you're switching directly from an aluminum-based commercial brand deodorant. The aluminum in antiperspirant deodorant actually keeps you from sweating by blocking your pores. When you stop using that deodorant, it gives your body a chance to cleanse itself. Unfortunately, that means months and months of backed-up toxins are now going to come out.

Allow your body to detox—that's why we have armpits, after all. You can help the process along by scrubbing your underarms with a shower brush and putting in extra work hours so you sweat more.

You'll also begin to notice that some days, you don't stink at all while other days, you stink a whole lot. This is mainly based on what you put into your body during the day. The more processed and toxin-filled foods and drinks that you consume, the stinkier you're going to be. So, if you're ditching the antiperspirant, ditch the fake food too!

Here are two deodorants—one for the farm girl and the other for the farm fella. You can switch up the scents as you wish, but both deodorants contain tea tree essential oil, as it kills bad bacteria that may cause extra stink under those arms!

Farm Girl Deodorant

3 oz coconut oil

1.2 oz beeswax

.5 oz cocoa butter

¼ cup arrowroot powder (or baking soda, or combination of the two)

5 drops vitamin E oil

5 drops lavender essential oil

5 drops tea tree essential oil

3 drops peppermint essential oil

METHOD:

1. In a double boiler, mix together coconut oil, beeswax, and cocoa butter until completely melted.

2. Add in arrowroot powder/baking soda and mix well.

3. Turn off heat and add in vitamin E oil and essential oils. Combine completely.

4. Pour into deodorant containers and allow to cool before capping. Once cool, cap tightly, label, and store for up to one year. Use daily as necessary.

Note: To make this a "farm fella" deodorant, swap out the lavender and peppermint essential oils for cedarwood and cypress instead.

Shaving Cream

I've spent countless dollars on shaving cream. My husband has probably spent even more than I have. This quick and easy shaving cream can be made in just a few minutes, and it can even be tailored to your own needs and scent preference. This recipe specifically calls for tea tree essential oil, as it helps cleanse the pores and heals the skin. For this reason, it's perfect for the man who has acne break-outs on his face because of his commercial shaving cream, and it's helpful for the woman who can't stand razor bumps and nicks on her legs!

4 oz coconut oil

2 oz sweet almond oil

4 oz shea butter (or cocoa butter)

5 drops tea tree essential oil

3 drops eucalyptus essential oil

3 drops vetiver essential oil

METHOD:

1. In a double boiler, melt together coconut oil, almond oil, and shea butter. Put in a glass bowl and allow to cool completely.

2. With a stand mixer or hand mixer (or by hand), whip the mixture just as you would whip cream. As the mixture begins to whip up, add essential oils one drop at a time. You can add more or less of the essential oils, depending on your scent preference.

3. Store in a glass jar or tin and use within six months.

Chamomile Aftershave Lotion

Swap out the cedarwood and vetiver for lavender and tea tree for a more floral scent in this recipe. Play around with essential oils to create the scent you like the most!

.5 oz beeswax

4 oz sweet almond oil

4 oz chamomile tea

10 drops vitamin E

5 drops cedarwood essential oil

5 drops vetiver essential oil

3 drops peppermint essential oil

METHOD:

1. In a double boiler with a mason jar, add beeswax and sweet almond oil. Melt completely.

2. Remove the jar from the pan and allow it to cool to room temperature. The wax will begin hardening, making the oil cloudy-looking. If you waited too long, just melt it down again.

3. In a separate container combine chamomile tea, vitamin E, and essential oils together.

4. Slowly add the tea and essential oil mix to the oil/beeswax mix while using an immersion blender to whip it to a thick and creamy consistency.

5. Store in a closed container at room temperature for about two months (longer if refrigerated).

Herbal Toilet Spray

Toilet spray rose in popularity in the early 2000s when a company claimed that if you sprayed their magic product in the toilet bowl before using the bathroom, your you-know-what wouldn't stink. Well, this herbal toilet spray actually does work, and you can make it right at home and ditch the high-cost option. You can even toss it in your purse for when you're on the go! Shake the bottle, mist a few sprays into the toilet bowl, and go about your business. Don't forget to flush when you're done! Switch up the scents with multiple different oils, as long as there are always 20–25 drops of essential oil total.

1 tsp fractionated coconut oil

1 tsp rubbing alcohol

10 drops lemongrass essential oil

10 drops lavender essential oil

5 drops tea tree essential oil

¼ cup water

1- to 2-ounce glass spray bottle

METHOD:

1. In a 1- to 2-ounce glass spray bottle, combine coconut oil, alcohol, and essential oils.

2. Add water until bottle is full, leaving a headspace (about ¼ cup). Cap with sprayer. Shake well.

3. Before each use, shake well and then spray the toilet water a few times before you use the bathroom.

HERBAL ORAL HYGIENE

One of the first things I tossed out the window when I began my herbal journey was fluoride toothpaste. We still use it from time to time, because let's face it, we're human. But we try to use homemade tooth powder and coconut oil as often as possible. Not only is it healthier for you, but it also gets your teeth naturally white and clean, and maintains healthy oral hygiene.

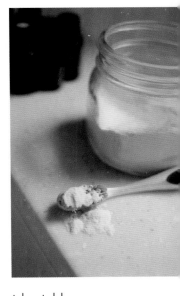

In our home we utilize a two-part system—tooth powder for brushing, and coconut oil for oil pulling. They really must go hand in hand to get the full benefit. If you don't know what "oil pulling" is, it's an ancient method practiced in India for more than three thousand years for healing the body. Today, we know that oil pulling is good for your teeth and your oral hygiene. Oils can literally pull plaque and impurities out of your teeth. Not only that, but it coats the teeth, giving them an extra barrier against new toxins and impurities that enter your body orally.

After brushing your teeth with the tooth powder (recipe below), swish a tablespoon of organic coconut oil in your mouth for twenty minutes. This not only naturally cleans your mouth, it pulls out any plaque and harsh bacteria that are still lurking there. It also naturally covers your teeth, repelling stains and food, keeping them squeaky clean throughout the day. Just make sure you don't rinse your mouth after oil pulling, as you can wash away all the beneficial oil that just coated your teeth!

If you can't make time for 20 minutes of oil pulling, 5–10 minutes is enough to coat the teeth and help seal them for the day. If you don't have time to oil pull at all, the tooth powder is fabulous on its own.

In this recipe, the baking soda naturally whitens and pulls out stains, the bentonite clay naturally pulls out toxins and decay from the teeth, the sea salt is a natural abrasive, and the peppermint cleans and freshens your breath. If you'd like to create an actual paste rather than a powder, simply mix all of these ingredients into softened organic coconut oil.

Peppermint Tooth Powder

1 cup baking soda

4–5 tbsp bentonite clay (or calcium carbonate)

1 tsp pink Himalayan sea salt (or regular sea salt)

1 tbsp diatomaceous earth

15 drops peppermint essential oil

METHOD:

1. In a glass jar, combine baking soda, diatomaceous earth, bentonite clay (or calcium carbonate), and salt. Mix well.

2. Add essential oils and mix until completely combined.

3. Cap, label, and store in your bathroom until ready for the next batch.

4. To use, simply dip your wet toothbrush into the mixture and brush as usual. There won't be any bubbles, but your mouth will naturally create a paste. Rinse mouth out well.

HERBAL LOTION BARS

A lot of people love lotion, but need some extra TLC when it comes to skin care. That's where lotion bars come in. They have all the healthy benefits of lotion, but instead of just soaking directly into the skin, they also seal in that moisture since they are beeswax based. You simply rub the lotion bar on a dry area of the skin that needs extra attention. This works well for rough elbows, heels and feet, and knees. Lotion bars look a lot like soap, but aren't used in the same way. However, the awesome part is that lotion bars are ten times easier to make than soap bars! This particular recipe makes 2–4 bars, depending on your mold size.

Skin-Healing Lavender and Calendula Lotion Bars

½ oz lavender-infused oil

½ oz calendula-infused oil

1 oz cocoa butter

1 oz beeswax

METHOD:

1. In a double boiler, combine all ingredients until completely melted.

2. Pour into square molds or a muffin pan. Allow to cool until completely hard (a couple of hours).

3. Pop bars out, wrap in paper or put in a sealed container, and label. Use within one year.

Chamomile and Honey Soothing Lotion Bars

1 oz chamomile-infused oil

1 oz cocoa butter

1 oz beeswax

1 tbsp raw honey

METHOD:

1. In a double boiler, combine infused oil, cocoa butter, and beeswax until completely melted.

2. Remove from heat and quickly mix in raw honey.

3. Pour into square molds or a muffin pan. Allow to cool until completely hard (a couple of hours).

4. Pop bars out, wrap in paper or put in a sealed container, and label. Use within 6–8 months.

Citrus and Mint Lotion Bars

If you don't want to use peppermint in this recipe, swap out the sweet almond oil with a spearmint-infused oil.

1 oz sweet almond oil

1 oz shea butter

1 oz beeswax

5 drops tangerine essential oil

3 drops peppermint essential oil

METHOD:

1. In a double boiler, combine oil, shea butter, and beeswax until completely melted.

2. Remove from heat and quickly add essential oils. Mix well.

3. Pour into square molds or a muffin pan. Allow to cool until completely hard (a couple of hours).

4. Pop bars out, wrap in paper or put in a sealed container, and label. Use within one year.

Pain-Soothing Lotion Bars

This lotion bar is great to keep on hand for aching skin, though not necessarily broken skin. It's especially great for feet that are aching after a long day.

½ oz cayenne-infused sweet almond oil

½ oz arnica-infused sweet almond oil

1 oz shea butter

1 oz beeswax

METHOD:

1. In a double boiler, combine all ingredients until completely melted.

2. Pour into square molds or a muffin pan. Allow to cool until completely hard (a couple of hours).

3. Pop bars out, wrap in paper or put in a sealed container, and label. Use within one year.

Herbs for lotion bars

Try these skin-healing herbs in your lotion bar, either as infused oils or in essential oil form (or both!).

Plantain	Chamomile	Lemongrass
Calendula	Lavender	Turmeric
Comfrey	Burdock	Rose

HOW TO MAKE SIMPLE SOAPS

I have yet to master the art of soapmaking at the Fewell homestead. There, I said it. It's just one of those things where I usually throw money at my homestead friends and hope they'll throw back a bar of soap. They haven't let me down yet. In fact, bartering works just as well. *Here, have a chicken. Thanks for the soap!*

But before I get to the recipes, I can take you through the rundown on soap-making basics.

Using lye. Yeah, lye. You know, that stuff that could potentially burn your eyes out, not the lie you tell your spouse when you bring home twenty new chickens instead of five. While it can absolutely be harmful and should be respected (the lye, not your chicken-buying impulse), it's also a necessary component for creating soap. And no, you can't make soap without lye, unless you're using a premade meltable soap base, which already has lye in it.

Lye doesn't have to be intimidating. It is simply a chemical made from salt, also known as sodium hydroxide. Lye is a necessary chemical to create soap because it reacts with the other ingredients to bind everything together**. After the soap has cured, the lye is completely gone from the soap,** as are the other oils, and you're left with a beautiful brick of pure, natural soap.

Important lye safety
It is very important to be safe when using lye!

Always add the lye into the water, **not** the water into the lye!

Do not use aluminum utensils or bowls when using lye, as it causes harmful fumes.

Never leave lye unattended once it's poured into a mixture.

Keep lye locked away out of the reach of children and animals.

If you should get lye on your skin, immediately wash thoroughly.

Always make soap on a hard surface that is not easily melted away by lye. You can mix it in a bowl on top of a thick wooden cutting board, metal countertop, or even outside on the ground. In fact, making the mixture outside is often best so that the fumes aren't in your home.

Make sure you're near a source of water when mixing lye so that you can flush away the lye on your body should an accident occur.

Use thick plastic containers to make soap, as easily meltable containers will melt and leak.

Always use gloves and goggles during the lye-mixing process.

Seems like a lot of work to go through to get soap, doesn't it? But I promise, it is very much worth it if you're trying to get away from chemical-laden soaps from the store that are packed full of preservatives and unnatural things for the skin. Also, most recipes for soap create a large batch all at one time. In other words, you shouldn't have to make soap very often if you make several batches at once.

Using lard (pig fat) instead of oils. I love lard, man. Slap that stuff in a cast-iron skillet and get 'er done. But lard can also be used in soap in place of coconut oil and other oils. In fact, it was most commonly used throughout the past few centuries because it was more readily available. Not only is it healthy and a way to get rid of waste, it's also a lot less expensive if you already have lard on hand from your recent pig processing rather than going out and buying oils. You can also use tallow, which is rendered cow fat. Unfortunately, lard doesn't lather very well, so I would suggest adding another oil, such as castor, along with lard into your recipe.

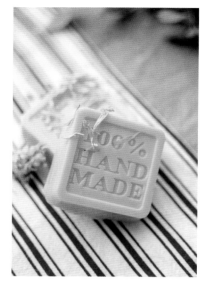

Hot processing versus cold processing. Well, I confess I didn't know there were even two types of soap processing until I walked over to my neighbor's house one day and she said, "Are you making hot- or cold-processed soap?" *Ummm, come again?* Apparently, you need to know this. Apparently, I needed to know this. Yes, my friend, there is a difference.

The major difference, without getting too far into it (I included an awesome book in the "Resources" chapter), is that cold-processed soaps (the recipes in this book) take 4–6 weeks to cure, whereas hot-processed soaps are cured by heat (usually in a crockpot) until all of the lye is cooked out. You can use the hot-processed soap after a few days. Unfortunately, it's a softer soap, and doesn't lend well to designs and molds.

SIMPLE SOAPMAKING ON THE HOMESTEAD

Most soapmaking recipes are similar in technique but differ in ingredients. Let's learn how to master the technique, and then I'll give you the ingredient lists for each different type of soap.

The ingredients for most soap recipes are the same:

  lye

  distilled water (or floral/herbal tea)

Caution

Before you begin, make sure you have on your protective eye gear and gloves!

solid fats (coconut oil, lard, or butters like shea and cocoa—these can be herbally infused)

liquid fats (olive oil, castor oil—these can also be herbally infused)

Soapmaking Method

Step 1: Make the lye solution

Carefully stir the lye (sodium hydroxide) into the distilled water (or herbal tea) until dissolved (never the other way around!). You can use construction-grade plastic containers or glass containers to mix the lye in. Work in an area with good ventilation and be careful not to breathe in the fumes. Outside in a covered area works well. The lye solution will get extremely hot, so set it aside to cool for about 30–40 minutes or until the temperature drops to around 100°F–110°F (38°C–43°C) on a meat or infrared thermometer.

Step 2: Prepare the solid oils, fats, and butters

Gently heat the solid oils and fats on low heat until melted. When the solid oils are melted, take the pan off the heat and pour into the liquid oil(s). This helps cool down the melted oil and fat, while warming up the room-temperature oil.

If you want to add powdered milk to your soap, blend it into the oils at this point.

Add this to your soaps!

½ tbsp powdered milk (cow, goat, coconut), stirred into the oils before adding the cooled lye solution

1 tbsp finely ground oats, stirred into the soap before pouring into the mold

1 tsp honey diluted with 1 tsp water, stirred into the soap before pouring into the mold

Step 3: Mixing

Pour the cooled lye solution into the warm oils. Using a combination of hand stirring and an immersion blender, also called a stick blender, stir the soap batter until it thickens and reaches trace (see sidebar).

If you plan to add honey and oats, blend them in at this stage.

Step 4: Pour into molds

Pour the mixed soap batter into your soap molds. Cover your soap-filled molds lightly with wax or freezer paper, then place a towel or light blanket over the top for insulation. Check the soap every so often to ensure it is cooling properly. If it begins to crack, uncover and move the soap to a cooler location.

Step 5: Cut and cure

Your brand new soap is safe to touch without gloves 48 hours after making it, but it needs the extra time to allow excessive moisture to evaporate so that the bars are harder and last longer.

Keep the soap in the molds for 1–2 days or until it's easy to remove, then slice it into bars when it's firm enough to not stick to your cutting tool. If you're using individual molds, simply pop them out when ready. Cure on coated cooling racks or sheets of wax paper for about four weeks before using.

THE RECIPES

Seeing as I'm no expert in soapmaking , I've roped my friend Jan Berry, author of *Simple & Natural Soapmaking* and blogger over at The Nerdy Farm Wife, into sharing a few of her herb soap recipes. You can take these basic recipes and make them your very own with herbs, essential oils, and more!

What is "trace"?

Trace is when the soap has thickened enough so that when you drizzle a small amount of the batter across the surface, it will leave a faint but visible imprint, or "trace," before sinking back in. This can take anywhere from 2–8 minutes, depending on how warm your ingredients are and how much you stir.

Basic Soap Recipe

OILS AND BUTTERS:

14 oz (397 g) olive oil (50%)

8.5 oz (241 g) coconut oil (30%)

4.5 oz (128 g) sunflower oil (16%)

1 oz (28 g) castor oil (4%)

LYE SOLUTION:

3.95 oz (112 g) lye

9 oz (255 g) distilled water

OPTIONAL EXTRAS:

30–35 g essential oils (like lavender, vetiver, chamomile, and more)

Old-Fashioned Lard Soap

OILS AND BUTTERS:

10 oz (283 g) olive oil (36%)

7.5 oz (213 g) coconut oil (27%)

4 oz (113 g) sunflower oil (14%)

6.5 oz (184 g) lard/tallow (23%)

LYE SOLUTION:

3.95 oz (112 g) lye

9 oz (255 g) distilled water

OPTIONAL EXTRAS:

30–35 g essential oils

Chamomile-Lavender Soap

OILS AND BUTTERS:

14 oz (397 g) olive oil (50%)

8.5 oz (241 g) chamomile-infused coconut oil (30%)

4.5 oz (128 g) sunflower oil (16%)

1 oz (28 g) castor oil (4%)

LYE SOLUTION:

3.95 oz (112 g) lye

9 oz (255 g) lavender tea

AT LIGHT TRACE:

10 g lavender essential oil

Simple Shea Butter Soap

OILS AND BUTTERS:

13 oz (369 g) olive oil (46%)

8 oz (227 g) coconut oil (29%)

5 oz (142 g) shea butter (18%)

2 oz (57 g) castor oil (7%)

LYE SOLUTION:

3.90 oz (111 g) lye

9 oz (255 g) distilled water

OPTIONAL EXTRAS:

30–35 g essential oils

Plantain Aloe Soap

OILS AND BUTTERS:

13 oz (369 g) olive oil (46.5%)

7.5 oz (213 g) plantain-infused coconut oil (27%)

4 oz (113 g) sunflower oil (14%)

2 oz (57 g) hemp oil (7%)

1.5 oz (43 g) castor oil (5.5%)

LYE SOLUTION:

3.95 oz (112 g) lye

6.5 oz (184 g) distilled water

2 oz (57 g) aloe liquid

¼ tsp chlorella powder (for color)

Create your own!

Use these simple recipes and substitute oils, fats, and milks that are infused with herbs like chamomile, plantain, calendula, and more. Add essential oils at light trace in all these recipes to enhance the scent!

Simple Goat's Milk Soap

OILS AND BUTTERS:

15 oz (425 g) olive oil

7 oz (198 g) coconut oil

2 oz (57 g) castor oil

2 oz (57 g) rice bran oil (or olive oil)

2 oz (57 g) sweet almond oil
(or sunflower oil)

LYE SOLUTION:

3.91 oz (111 g) lye

4 oz (113 g) distilled water (or infused tea)

4 oz (113 g) goat's milk (or infused goat's milk)

OPTIONAL EXTRAS:

20–30 g essential oils added at light trace

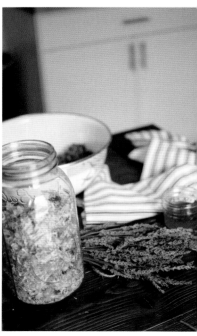

Out of all the health and beauty creations you can make with herbs, soap may be the most complicated of them all, but have full confidence that practice makes perfect. Start simple, with things like lotion bars and toothpaste, and then eventually work your way up to the more complicated creations. When you feel confident enough, use the herb list in the beginning of this book (chapter 2) as a guide to help you master your own personalized herbal health products.

I am always amazed by how easy it is to make the herbal alternative to the products that we use in everyday life. It takes me less time to create a lip balm or shaving cream than it does for me to drive to the store. This is just one of the numerous reasons that I try to create so many of our own products because—let's face it—more time in the day is never a bad thing! And who really likes going to the grocery store?

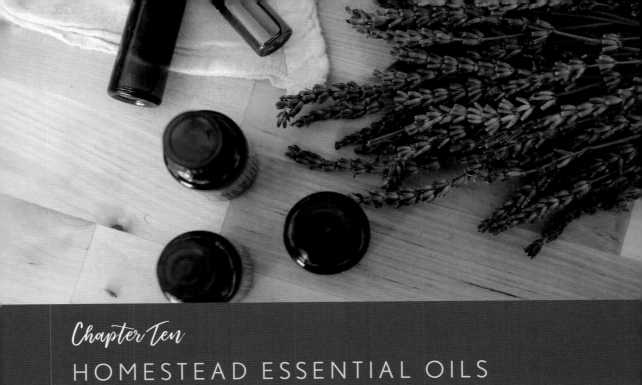

Chapter Ten

HOMESTEAD ESSENTIAL OILS

Chances are if you're reading this book, you don't think essential oils are just something con artists claim will cure all your ailments, like snake oil. Essential oils have been used for centuries. That's right, centuries. As far back as the Egyptians, we know that essential oils were used for various purposes such as mummification and healing. Essential oils aren't a new fad at all; they are simply becoming popular again.

But what are they exactly? Essential oils are naturally occurring volatile aromatic compounds found in the seeds, bark, stems, roots, flowers, and other parts of plants. They protect plants against environmental threats and provide beneficial properties to the plant and to those of us who use them. They are highly concentrated when distilled for purity and potency, oftentimes taking several pounds of plant matter to create one small bottle of essential oil.

With just a few drops of oil, you can have a potent and efficient remedy through topical, aromatic, or ingested application of an herb via essential oils. Essential

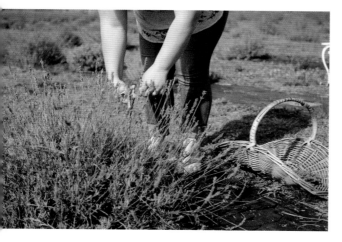

oils are great for general health and ailments, but we also really enjoy using them on the homestead for cleaning and aromatic purposes.

It's not necessarily economical to make your own essential oils, though many herbalists do, so I'm not going to cover that here. Instead I will focus on their use. There are a few trusted companies that I enjoy buying from. Be aware that there are many big-box stores and online retail sources that sell millions of different products not related to essential oils. They are typically not as pure or safe.

That's a lot of lavender!

It takes roughly 3 pounds (lbs) of lavender to make a 15-milliliter (mL) bottle of lavender essential oil. It takes roughly 63 lbs of lemon balm to make a 5 mL bottle of essential oil.

Essential oils aren't cheap or easy to make, but they are absolutely worth purchasing. If you're in the mood, eventually, you might even try making your own with a distillery system.

I most often like to use essential oils on my homestead when I need a quick fix. We use essential oils aromatically, topically, and sometimes we ingest them. Essential oils are great to help treat common ailments, clean and heal wounds, reduce headaches, uplift the spirit, clean the home and barn, and purify the air.

The Egyptians were some of the earliest users of essential oils, though their oils weren't identical to the types of oils we use today. Egyptians would often use animal fats and oils to infuse herbs into oils. Hydrodistillation of herbs to create essential oils didn't really begin until the ancient Greeks, around 1850 BC. They distilled essential oils from plants like rosemary, coriander, and lavender. Often, they used essential oils aromatically to enhance sleep, boost mood, and purify the air. They used them antiseptically, and even diffused them into the air during times of plague and sickness.

Throughout the Old Testament and Torah, we learn that the ancient people of Israel used essential oils extensively as aromatics, in balms and salves, and incense. In fact, they brought herbal gifts of frankincense and myrrh to Jesus when He was born, and spikenard was often used for anointing people during prayer.

Essential oils didn't really begin to come back into popularity until the mid-nineteenth century and were mainly used as aromatics and in cosmetics and beauty products. We still use essential oils in cosmetics and beauty products today, though not necessarily therapeutic grade oils.

My favorite essential oils

Tea Tree	Lemongrass
Thyme	Lavender
Oregano	Peppermint
Lemon Balm	Clary Sage
Vetiver	Frankincense
Ylang Ylang	

With the help of modern science, we've discovered that essential oils can be used more than just aromatically. With guidance, they can be ingested and can even help the body's healing process, and promote general good health. However, there is a proper way and an improper way to use them. With most new products, we are often quick to use them on anything and everything. Remember the antibiotic resistance issue? Let's not do with essential oils what we did with antibiotics.

HOW TO USE ESSENTIAL OILS

There are a few different ways to use essential oils, but we should always exercise caution. The typical dosage of oils for an adult is 2–3 drops for aromatic and topical application. Let's go over the ways in which to use essential oils most effectively.

Things to know about essential oils (EOs)

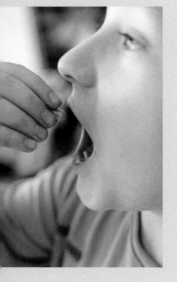

- Always use a carrier oil on sensitive skin, children, or with "hot" oils (like peppermint, oregano, and basil).

- It's best to ingest EOs through a capsule, in honey, or on a sugar cube, not in a drink, as most of the oil is lost on the sides of the glass. A raw essential oil can cause harm to the stomach lining.

- A little goes a long way. Always start with less rather than more.

- Do your research extensively before using EOs on an infant or those who are pregnant or nursing.

- Some EOs should not be used on people who have certain autoimmune disorders, seizures, diabetes, or other diseases. Please do your research or consult a physician first.

- When applying EOs, apply directly to the portion of the body that needs attention, or use the reflex points on your feet and hands.

Topical Application

Topical application is the most-often used method of administering essential oils. If you have sensitive skin, are administering to a child, or are using a hot oil, you'll need to use a carrier oil before applying the essential oil. You can do this by putting the carrier oil on first and then the essential oil, or you can simply make a blend in a small dish with carrier oil and essential oil. If you do not have sensitive skin and you're not using a hot oil, many oils can be applied directly to the skin. My two favorite carrier oils are jojoba oil and fractionated coconut oil.

Other ways to apply topically:

Compresses. Fill a large bowl or wash basin with hot, but not boiling, water. Add essential oils (3–4 drops) to the water and stir vigorously. Lay a small hand rag or

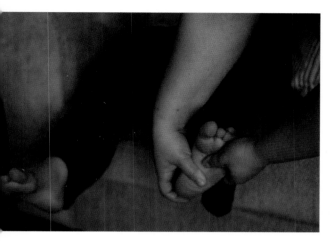

towel on top of the water to absorb the oils and some of the water. When the rag/towel is completely saturated, wring out the towel and place it on the part of the body that needs attention. Cover with a dry towel to help hold in the heat. You can also make cold compresses, especially during times of inflammation or summer heat. Simply switch out the hot water for cold water.

Massage Therapy. Making essential oil blends with carrier oil and essential oils for massage therapy works wonders. Simply blend your carrier oil with your desired essential oils in a large glass bottle, shake well, and directly apply to the body while massaging reflex points. (See the essential oil blend recipes in this chapter.)

Roll-On Bottles. Sometimes you might be on the go and need an extra boost or need your oils to reduce headaches, inflammation, or bug bites. This is where roll-on bottles come in handy. Simply place the essential oils of your choice in a glass roll-on bottle and fill up the remaining portion of the bottle with carrier oil. Shake well before each use, concentrating on reflex points for application or applying directly to the spot of pain or discomfort.

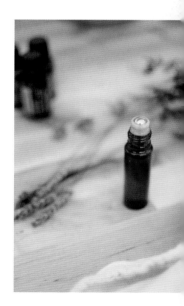

Make Your Own Blends

You can make your very own blends of essential oils for topical use or for roll-on bottles. This is one of the most efficient ways to take advantage of multiple oils that have similar uses. Simply add drops of the oils to a roll-on bottle or new essential oil bottle, then fill the remaining portion of the bottle with carrier oil. I typically only use 1-ounce bottles to make blends, as they begin to lose their potency once blended with a carrier oil. Use up these blends within six months.

Headache Blend: Use this blend to help reduce stress and tension headaches.

Peppermint • Frankincense • Lavender

Respiratory Blend: The perfect blend for allergy season, respiratory infections and colds, or when you need open airways.

Peppermint • Eucalyptus (E. radiata) • Tea Tree (Melaleuca alternifolia) • Clove

Women's Blend: This blend saves me every month. It's perfect for hormonal balance, thyroid function, and overall monthly "time of the month" comfort.

Clary Sage • Bergamot • Ylang Ylang • Geranium • Tangerine • Cinnamon Bark

Digestive Blend: When you've eaten too much at Thanksgiving, or when your body needs extra digestive aid, this is the blend to rub on your tummy or ingest by capsule.

Ginger • Peppermint • Fennel • Lavender

"I've Got Joy" Blend: I've got the joy, joy, joy, joy down in my heart. *Where?* I remember singing that joyful song when I was a kid, and now it gets to spill over into this joyful blend! Use this blend when you need emotional support or you're just feeling down and tired.

Lavender • Tangerine • Lemongrass • Lemon Balm (Melissa) • Ylang Ylang • Hawaiian Sandalwood

Immune-Boosting Blend: This blend is best put on the bottoms of the feet in the evenings before going to bed. Use this blend to boost immunity and help your body fight colds and general sickness.

Clove • Cinnamon Bark • Eucalyptus (E. radiata) • Rosemary • Oregano • Tea Tree

Wound Healing Blend: This blend has taken the place of peroxide or rubbing alcohol in our house when it comes to cleaning out wounds. Use this blend to clean and heal wounds more quickly—for humans *and* animals!

Tea Tree • Oregano • Lavender • Helichrysum

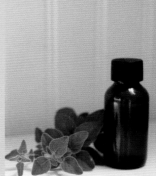

Sleepytime Blend: When the little ones need some extra comfort and encouragement to fall asleep or when you just need to promote a sense of rest—use this. Just do it. Use topically or aromatically.

Lavender • Roman Chamomile • Vetiver • Cedarwood • Ylang Ylang • Marjoram

Purifying Blend: Toss this blend into soiled clothing in the wash. Diffuse it in the air during times of sickness. Whatever you do, this blend helps cleanse and purify.

Lemon • Lime • Tea Tree • Cilantro • White Fir

Bug-Repelling Blend: I'm not sure where we would be without this blend. It saves our legs from mass attacks by mosquitoes in the summer months—the perfect bug-repelling blend! Put into a spray bottle with witch hazel or simply make a blend to use directly on the skin with carrier oil.

Ylang Ylang • Cedarwood • Citronella • Lemongrass • Eucalyptus • Arborvitae • Catnip

Using Essential Oils Aromatically

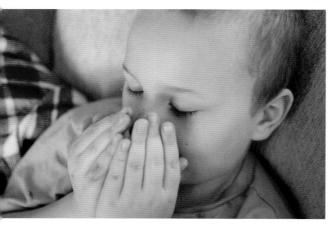

If you were to ask certain herbalists, they would tell you that essential oils should only be used aromatically. This is simply because it has been taught this way through folk and generational habits. Through modern science, we know that there are right and wrong ways to use essential oils, but that they can also be used more than just as aromatics alone.

With that said, essential oils are still powerful via scent. They can be used to purify the air, treat symptoms of depression and anxiety (like diffusing the *I've Got Joy* blend), and reduce inflammation in the airways, and they are a fantastic alternative to chemical-filled candles and air fresheners.

Using an Electric Diffuser. You can purchase a diffuser from your local store or online. Each electric diffuser is different, but they all have the same concept.

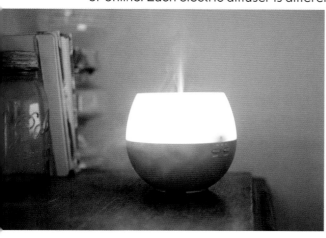

Simply fill your diffuser up with the proper water amount. Add 2–4 drops of your essential oil or blend to the top of the water. Place the cap back on the diffuser, turn on, and place in an area of the room where it will be most beneficial. Most diffusers will fill up an entire standard-size room. For larger, more open rooms, they may only reach part of the room. We use a diffuser in the wintertime to purify the air, help with respiratory distress, clear the airways, and around the holidays as a natural air freshener.

Reed Diffuser

If you're off the grid or simply don't want to use an electric diffuser, you can create an old-fashioned reed diffuser just as easily.

reeds or bamboo sticks (chopsticks work, too)

vodka, rubbing alcohol, or witch hazel

distilled water

essential oils

vase, crock, or mason jar

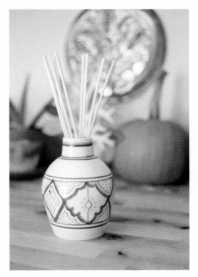

METHOD:

1. In your container (vase, etc.), add 1 part distilled water and 1 part liquid (vodka, witch hazel, or rubbing alcohol).

2. Add in 4–6 drops of your essential oil or blend and mix well.

3. Place reeds/bamboo sticks in the liquid and allow to absorb for 15 minutes.

4. Flip reeds/bamboo sticks over, placing the dry end in the liquid.

Note: You now have a reed diffuser. The scent travels up the stick and fills the air. When the scent begins to dissipate (in a couple of days), simply flip the reeds over again. Use until liquid is gone, then make a new batch!

Using Essential Oils Internally

Ingest them. Don't ingest them. Ingest them a certain way. There is a constant debate about ingesting essential oils, but there's really nothing black and white about it. For years we were told not to ingest essential oils, then we transitioned

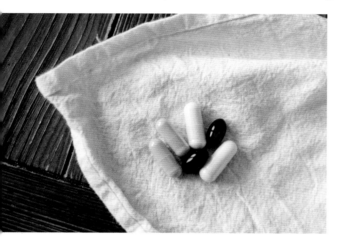

to a period of time where we ingested them frequently. It's like being told that we should eat butter, and then that we shouldn't. Or that coconut oil is healthy for us, but then ten years later, it's not. Newsflash: I'm not getting rid of either! Especially not my butter. Amen.

As with everything, there is a fine balance with ingesting essential oils, and I prefer to tackle it from a scientific standpoint.

Essential oils shouldn't be ingested on a regular basis unless there is a good reason for doing so—inflammation, headaches, digestive issues, certain diseases, etc. Taking essential oils internally for an extended period of time is never recommended unless it has been advised by a certified professional. Think about it, we don't even ingest herbs in their natural form for longer than eight weeks in medicinal doses, so why would we ingest essential oils longer than that? And essential oils are exactly that—medicinal doses.

There's a big difference between using essential oils topically and ingesting them. They can be much more detrimental when ingested. Please do your research on which oils can and cannot be ingested. And make sure you always ingest them with food, honey, or in a capsule, never in a drink.

Essential oils can absolutely be used in cooking and to enhance the flavors of things. This is okay because the oil is being used in a product, not on its own. Just 1–3 drops will do the trick when cooking or baking with essential oils, and the flavor is incomparably delicious. Just keep in mind that essential oils, when cooked at high heat, lose all of their medicinal properties, so you're essentially just using them as flavoring.

DISTILLING YOUR OWN ESSENTIAL OILS

So, you want to make your own essential oils. I get it, I really do. I would love to try my hand at it. I've had my eye on a copper distiller for some time now, but mainly because it's just pretty. I don't think I can convince my husband we need one just because it's pretty, though.

Unfortunately, I don't have endless amounts of herbs on my homestead. I suppose I could purchase 3 pounds of lavender to make a 15-milliliter bottle of lavender essential oil, but—have you priced lavender lately? I'd literally be spending hundreds, possibly thousands, of dollars just for the lavender when I can buy pure lavender essential oil from my favorite essential oil company for $20.

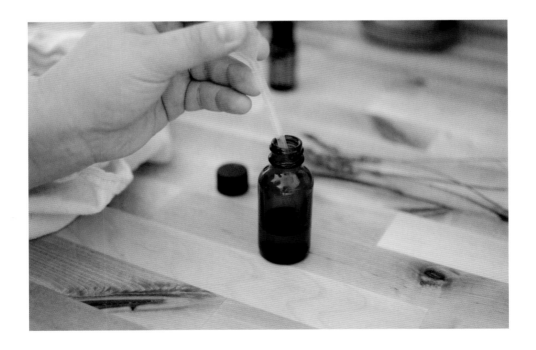

With that said, you can most certainly make your own essential oils in small batches. This is especially true for people who own large farms with ample amounts of herbs, or for those who are simply science geeks, like me.

To begin, you'll need a distiller. Think "moonshine." It's the same exact concept. You heat up your herb, and the herb condenses and separates the oils from the water. And eventually you're left with a beautiful essential oil at the end of the process.

You can purchase distillers online or from local sources that make them by hand, although you might have to convince your local sheriff that you aren't up to any funny business should he come knockin'.

Keep in mind that your end product may not be as pure as commercial distilled essential oils. With large commercial distillers in sanitized areas, this is one of those things I typically leave to the pros. More likely than not, you won't be able to create enough high heat to burn off any unwanted solvent that's left in your solution. But you can certainly try!

Once you've gotten your distiller, you'll need to follow the instructions that came with it. Each distiller is different, and my telling you how to do it exactly in this book may just get you hurt. Please be safe and read the directions first.

You can see from the illustration just how a distiller works. Because plants are mostly water, the oils have to be extracted through high heat, evaporated, and then formed into the oil. This is an incredibly fun adult science experiment, and people have been making essential oils for centuries this way. Take your time, enjoy the process, and the end result will bring so much satisfaction.

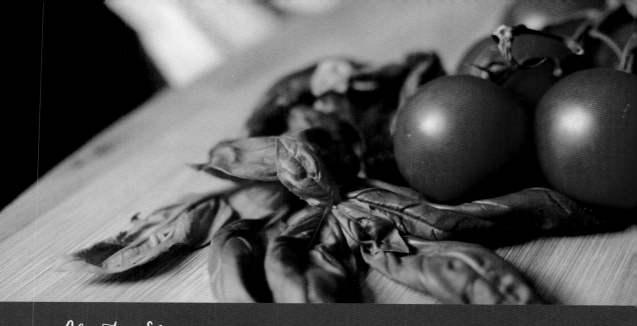

Chapter Eleven
COOKING WITH HERBS ON THE HOMESTEAD

My husband loves to eat. I love to eat. My kid loves to eat. My chickens love to eat what we don't eat. My dogs love to eat what I want to eat so much that they sneak it off of my plate. We love food. Period. Especially good, wholesome, homemade food.

When you run a homestead, eating is mandatory. Fresh produce and herbs from the garden, a grass-fed beef steak sitting on the kitchen countertop, and a cast-iron skillet, hot and ready and full of butter on the burner—this is what dreams are made of. Well, at least my dreams.

This is my place of solitude. This is where we live. I often tell my husband that I don't care how big or small the bedrooms are in our house, give me a gigantic farmhouse kitchen and dining area (and herb garden!) and I'll live a happy life forever.

We literally live and breathe in our farmhouse kitchen. All of our meals, harvests, preservation, and joys happen in the midst of these four walls. Life breathes into us, and we breathe it back out with herbs and spices lingering on our breath—the kind of herbs that give us life, joy, and good food in our bellies; the kind of herbs that enhance the bounty of vegetables, homegrown or hunted meat, and even the glass of wine you drink while cooking. Growing up, I used to make random food creations in our family kitchen. I'd act like I was Julia Child, making recipes from other countries like France and Italy. Somehow I thought that roasting a chicken with thyme and rosemary was something extravagant. Now it's just normal, everyday life for me. But I still haven't forgotten the excitement I had when I first mastered roasted chicken.

Now that I've grown up and have a family of my own, I try my best to make my creations as palatable as possible. Thankfully, I'm succeeding, and herbs have made my cooking more exciting. In fact, I've discovered that when you use herbs to season your food instead of just salt, you often don't need that much salt to begin with and your food tastes so much better and is healthier for your family.

These are the herbs that I keep very close by on a regular basis. While my culinary herb collection is extensive, I often find myself grabbing for these, sometimes even when a recipe doesn't call for it. In fact, Julia Child said it best herself when

My favorite (and most often used) culinary herbs.

Thyme	Cilantro	Turmeric	Clove
Oregano	Rosemary	Bay Leaf	Parsley
Garlic	Sage	Cumin	Curry
Onion	Basil	Cinnamon	Dill

she told us that learning how to cook from scratch means you aren't enslaved to recipes. Whatever grows in season, you know exactly what to do with it. And she was absolutely right.

When you've been cooking with herbs for a while, you find that you don't always stick to the recipe; you go more by smell and taste. Instinct is what they call it, I suppose. You begin to know which aromas go with which herbs, which herbs enhance which meats, and so on.

I always chuckle when I have successfully prepared a meal completely from scratch and my husband, Mark, insists that someone else created the recipe, not me. It could be partly because I really didn't know how to cook when we first got married. Or it could be partly because he's giving me a hard time, like he usually does. One can never tell. I just kiss him and make him smile.

Herbs and growing our own food on this homestead have taught me how to cook. There's a newfound love for cooking that comes when you grow something with your own two hands, in the very dirt you walk on, with the very heart from which you loved and nurtured it.

PAIRING HERBS WITH MEATS

My husband Mark is an avid hunter. I'd like to think I could be too, but he never takes me. It's his place of solitude, just as my kitchen is mine.

While my grandfather often hunted, I never really tried much venison growing up. But now it has become one of my favorite things to cook. And trust me, it is available in abundance along this Virginia mountainside all year long. It's true that you haven't had good venison until you've cooked and seasoned it properly. When it's cooked medium-rare with the proper herbs, and allowed to rest for five minutes before serving, it will make your stomach happy.

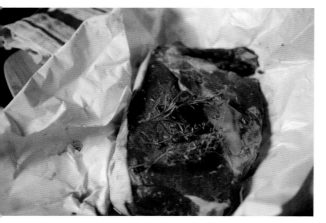

My second runner-up would have to be grass-fed beef. My sister-in-law and her husband sure do know how to "grow" a good slab of beef, and we gladly reap the benefits of their labor. It's tender, juicy, and full of natural flavor. And it pairs well with a mean dish of mashed potatoes and garlic, and homemade bread and butter.

Of course, I love roasted chicken, too. I love food, remember? And I'm going to teach you how to make that roasted chicken in just a bit. But first, let's learn which herbs pair best with which meats. My general rule is, when in doubt, keep it simple.

Venison: bay leaf, thyme, rosemary, garlic, onion, sage, juniper berries, cayenne

Beef: rosemary, thyme, garlic, onion, bay leaf, cayenne

Chicken: garlic, thyme, turmeric, parsley, curry, oregano, rosemary, tarragon, sage, onion, basil, cayenne

Rabbit: garlic, bay leaf, curry, onion, parsley, rosemary, thyme, saffron, coriander, marjoram, juniper berries

Quail: bay leaf, garlic, mint, sage, thyme, onion

Pork: marjoram, cinnamon, mustard, sage, oregano, thyme, rosemary, garlic

Fish: garlic, thyme, rosemary, oregano, lovage, sorrel

Duck: marjoram, rosemary, saffron, sage, tarragon, thyme, curry, turmeric, paprika, parsley, juniper berries

Turkey: basil, rosemary, thyme, cumin, sage, cayenne

THE RECIPES

Now for the good stuff. What's an herb book without a few recipes from the kitchen, right? Being an herbal homesteader isn't just about living a healthy lifestyle through herbs and herbal remedies, it's about enjoying the bounty you've harvested.

These are some of my very favorite recipes that my family has enjoyed time and thyme again (pun intended). And I am honored to share them with you because, not only have they been the very foundation of what has set my family on the path of wholesome eating, they have taught me how to use herbs to enhance flavor and experience.

Herb Spice Mix

This spice mix is my go-to for everything from roasted chicken to fried eggs and more! I season most dishes with it, even if it's just a pinch.

1 tbsp garlic powder

1 tbsp onion powder

1 tbsp paprika

1 tbsp thyme, dried

½ tbsp oregano, dried

½ tbsp turmeric powder

½ tbsp pepper

½ tsp chili powder

2 tsp salt

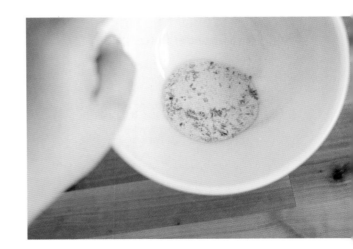

METHOD:

Mix all spices together in a jar to create an aromatic and simple herb spice mix. Use within a year.

Herbes de Provence

Most people often think of lavender when they think of Herbes de Provence, but lavender is not actually an original ingredient of this mix. Lavender in Herbes de Provence is more of a Westernized addition rather than a European tradition. The original Herbes de Provence recipe simply starts with rosemary, thyme, and bay leaf. You can add other types of herbs to enhance the flavor of whatever you may be cooking, such as dill, sage, and tarragon.

3½ tbsp thyme, dried

3 tsp rosemary, dried

2 tsp bay leaf, dried and crushed

1 tbsp oregano, dried

2 tbsp savory, dried

1 tsp marjoram, dried

2 tsp basil, dried

½ tsp fennel seed

1 tbsp lavender flowers, dried (optional)

METHOD:

Mix all herbs together and store in an airtight container in your pantry until ready to use. Use within a year.

Farmstead Roasted Chicken

I used to think making a roast chicken was complicated. Boy, was I wrong. This is the best roast chicken I've ever had in my entire life, though I could be quite biased. Either way, this chicken is sure to please. The real art of roasting a chicken isn't necessarily in the seasoning but in the roasting process and fluctuating temperatures. Keep this recipe simple and you'll have a crowd pleaser.

1 whole chicken (4–8 lbs)

4 tbsp butter, softened

1 tbsp herb spice mix (see recipe on page 207)

fresh rosemary and thyme (handfuls)

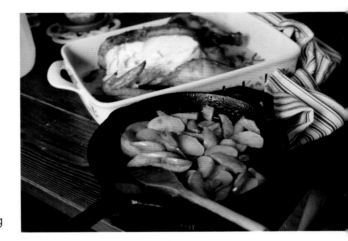

METHOD:

1. Preheat oven to 400°F.

2. Wash chicken thoroughly and pat dry with a paper towel. Place in baking dish.

3. With your hands, gently separate the skin from the breast portion of the chicken. Rub 2 tablespoons of softened butter underneath the skin, directly on the breast. Rub remaining portion of butter over the top of the skin all over until the entire bird is covered in butter.

4. Sprinkle herb spice mix evenly over the skin. You can sprinkle extra thyme and rosemary on as well.

5. Add handfuls of fresh rosemary and thyme into the cavity of the chicken.

6. Bake at 400°F for 30–40 minutes. Bring oven down to 375°F for the remaining 2 hours. Chicken is completely done when skin is crispy and brown and the temperature reaches 165°F on a meat thermometer inserted into the thickest part of the thigh. Your chicken will bake for a total of about 2½–3 hours.

Spicy Eggs, Bacon, and Kale

This dish is one of my favorite springtime lunches. We always have kale and fresh eggs in abundance during this time of year, and I'm always in need of ways to use them up quickly. This recipe does the trick.

slices of thick-cut bacon, roughly chopped (we use homegrown, no nitrates added)

1 small sweet onion, roughly chopped

3 garlic cloves, minced

2 bunches kale, de-stemmed and roughly chopped

1½ cup homemade chicken stock (see recipe on page xx)

8–10 quail eggs (or 4–5 farm fresh chicken eggs)

2 tsp black pepper

¼ tsp cayenne pepper

red pepper flakes, to taste

juice of 1 lemon

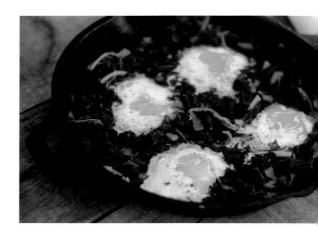

METHOD:

1. Fry bacon pieces in a large skillet (cast iron preferred) until crispy. Remove from skillet, leaving drippings.

2. Cook onions and garlic in drippings until opaque. Add additional oil if necessary.

3. Add bunches of kale, half at a time as space in skillet allows.

4. Add chicken stock and let simmer until kale is soft, about 5 minutes.

5. Create four small wells in the kale and crack one egg into each well.

6. Season entire mixture with black pepper, red pepper flakes, cayenne, and lemon juice.

7. Cover pan and allow eggs to cook until desired doneness. Turn off heat immediately, sprinkle on bacon, and serve.

Rustic Garlic and Chive Mashed Potatoes

Yes, I'm fully aware of how much butter is in this recipe. No, I don't care. Yes, you should use farm fresh, homemade raw butter if at all possible. Otherwise, purchase grass-fed butter. Yes, this recipe is amazing and to be indulged in occasionally, not every single night. Get it? Got it? Good.

5 lbs golden potatoes, rough chopped

5 cloves garlic

8 tbsp butter

4.5 oz cream cheese, softened

1–2 cups milk

salt and pepper, to taste

2 tbsp chives, fresh

METHOD:

1. In a large pot, place roughly chopped potatoes (leave skins on for a more rustic feel) and cover with water. You'll only need just enough water to cover them. Toss in five smashed garlic cloves as well. These will infuse the water and the potatoes. Boil for 20 minutes or until fork tender.

2. Drain potatoes and garlic. Mash potatoes and garlic together in a large bowl. If you don't want too much of a garlicky taste, only smash in two of the garlic cloves.

3. Add butter and cream cheese, cover with hot potato mash, and allow to melt for 3–5 minutes. Then mash your mixture together again. At this point, you can also use a hand blender for creamier texture.

4. Add milk until desired consistency.

5. Add salt and pepper to taste.

6. Add 1 tablespoon chives; mix well. Garnish the top with remaining chives. Serve it up and watch it disappear.

Thyme-Roasted Cherry Tomatoes, Potatoes, and Feta

Notice that I don't really measure in this recipe? You get to pick and choose how much of each ingredient you want to put in. The roasting process draws out the natural sweetness of the tomatoes against the twiggy thyme. This dish is best served warm, as the aromatics from the herbs and the warm feta really complement each other.

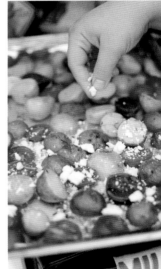

fingerling or baby potatoes, cut in half or rough chop

cherry tomatoes, cut in half

olive oil

2 tbsp fresh or dried thyme

salt and pepper

2 tsp herb spice mix (optional, see recipe on page 207)

fresh feta cheese

METHOD:

1. Spread potatoes and cherry tomatoes on a baking sheet. Drizzle with olive oil and toss potatoes and tomatoes to coat.

2. Season with thyme, salt, and pepper. You can even use the herb spice mix recipe.

3. Bake at 400°F degrees for 30 minutes or until potatoes are fork tender and tomatoes are completely roasted.

4. Sprinkle feta cheese over the potatoes and tomatoes and bake for 5–7 more minutes until feta is warm.

5. Serve warm for best flavor.

Simple Grass-fed Beef Steak

Grass-fed beef doesn't need an extravagant array of spices. The meat itself is flavorful and the herbs simply enhance its beefiness and aroma. Keep this simple, and you'll love yourself forever.

**garlic and rosemary herb butter
(see recipe on page 214)**

coarse salt and pepper

2–4 grass-fed beef steaks

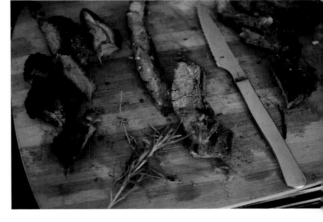

METHOD:

1. In a preheated cast-iron skillet, add 1–2 tablespoons of the garlic and rosemary herb butter.

2. Season steaks with salt and pepper, and lay them in preheated pan. Be careful not to crowd them.

3. Sear on the first side for 4–5 minutes. Turn once, and sear the second side for an additional 4 minutes, or until desired doneness. We like our steaks rare or medium rare, so this is a good time frame for a 1- to 2-inch steak.

4. Remove steak from pan and cover with tin foil. Place in the oven or set aside on a cutting board on the counter to finish cooking and to seal in the juices. Allow to rest for 8–10 minutes before cutting.

Herbed Butters

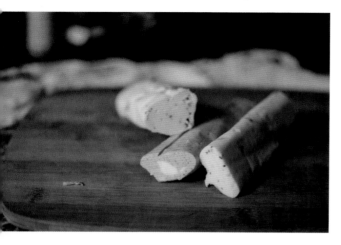

Adding herbs to butters is one of my favorite ways to use up fresh herbs in the summertime. They keep for quite a long time and they are great when you need to sear a steak, add a quick seasoning to a chicken dish, or just want to slather some on a thick piece of fresh bread. Use up butters made with fresh herbs within a couple of weeks. Butters made with dried herbs can last months. You can also freeze your butters for longer storage. They are extremely easy to make and are even more delicious when using your own homemade butter.

1 lb butter, softened, not melted

3–4 tbsp herbs of your choice, fresh or dried

METHOD:

1. Cut up herbs into small pieces or chop in a food processor.

2. Mix herbs and butter together thoroughly.

3. Roll into a log with parchment paper and keep in the refrigerator or freezer until ready to use. Slice off a piece of butter as necessary, or you can precut them into pieces and place them in a bag.

Some of my favorite combinations and what to use them on:

- **garlic and rosemary:** steaks, chicken, rabbit, quail, venison, pasta
- **lavender, thyme, and lemon zest:** biscuits, chicken, quail
- **honey and mint:** biscuits, bread, goat, chicken

- **garlic, chive, and pepper:** chicken, steak, rabbit, venison, focaccia
- **basil pesto:** pasta, focaccia, breads, chicken, steak
- **sage and lemon zest:** chicken, venison, pasta
- **parsley, lime, and cumin:** pasta, chicken, rice
- **cilantro and red pepper flakes:** chicken, rice
- **rosemary, orange zest, and thyme:** biscuits, bread, steak, chicken, rabbit, venison
- **thyme, oregano, and basil:** anything!

Traditional Rabbit Confit

I often like to call this "Lapin Confit." It's the traditional French name for "Rabbit Confit," and it just sounds so much more elegant than its American translation. But whether I'm in the French countryside or in my very own quaint Virginia countryside kitchen, this recipe is elegant and delicious either way.

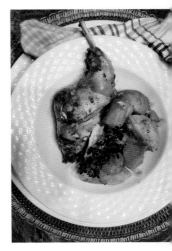

When we first started raising rabbits, this was one of the very first recipes I learned to make, and it never disappoints. I hope you enjoy it as much as I do. This recipe pairs well with the garlic mashed potatoes (see recipe on page 211) and the thyme roasted tomatoes (see recipe on page 212).

1 whole rabbit (or 4 rabbit thighs)

1 small yellow onion, roughly chopped

4 sprigs rosemary

5 garlic cloves

5 bay leaves, dried

1 heaping tbsp black peppercorns

10 sprigs thyme

1 tsp mustard seed

4 cardamom pods

salt and pepper, to taste

2–4 cups olive oil (or half oil and half melted lard)

METHOD:

1. Preheat oven to 275°F.

2. In a Dutch oven, add rabbit and all ingredients except oil/lard.

3. Add 2–4 cups of oil/lard, until the melted fat just about completely covers the rabbit. The rabbit will float. That's okay.

4. Cover the Dutch oven and place in the preheated oven for about 3 hours or until the rabbit is just about falling apart (but not yet!).

5. When done, remove the rabbit from the oil and place on a baking sheet. Pre-heat oven to 325°F. Cook the rabbit in the oven on the baking sheet until crisp. Don't overcook! Remember, the rabbit itself is already cooked.

6. Strain and reserve the oil from the Dutch oven to drizzle over the rabbit when ready to serve.

7. Pull the rabbit meat off of the bones, or cut the rabbit into pieces and serve warm with a drizzle of warm oil on top.

Grilled Herbed Pork Loin

If I had to choose a favorite way to put pork to good use, it would be with this recipe. I would admit that I could eat this entire loin myself, but I have to keep it classy. This recipe takes just a few minutes to make on the grill, and it will be your favorite dish to make all summer long. Just remember that pork doesn't have to be well done. A little bit of pink in the middle is the best way to eat homegrown pork.

1 pork loin

olive oil

½ tbsp herb mix seasoning
(see recipe on page 207)

½ tbsp rosemary

½ tbsp thyme

2 garlic cloves, minced

coarse salt and pepper, to taste

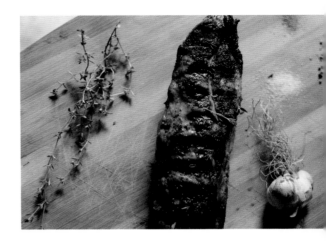

METHOD:

1. Cover entire loin with olive oil and rub down the loin with all of the herbs, garlic, salt, and pepper.

2. On a preheated grill or grill pan, use the 7-6-5 method to grill the loin. This means you grill the loin for 7 minutes on the first side, 6 minutes on the second side, flip the loin over one last time and turn the grill completely off, allowing it to rest for 5 minutes on the hot grill. The lid should remain closed at all times unless you're turning it. Make sure the internal temperature reaches 145°F or just under, as there will be a carryover cooking time period.

3. Remove from heat and allow to rest on a cutting board for 5–7 minutes.

4. Cut into medallions and serve warm with the juice that it releases as it rests (if any).

Goat Cheese, Spinach, and Herb Quiche

Heaven bless the person who looked at goat's milk and said, "This would make a wonderful cheese." Goat's milk cheese is my favorite of all the cheeses. It's tangy and creamy, and it pairs exceptionally well with herbs. This quiche is truly a farmer's quiche if you have goats, chickens, and an herb garden. This can be made from farm to table completely and easily. And, because this recipe isn't complete without the pie crust to go with it, I'll be nice and give you my pie crust recipe as well.

FOR THE PIE CRUST:

3 cups unbleached flour

1 cup cold salted butter

1 large egg

⅓ cup cold water

1 tbsp apple cider vinegar

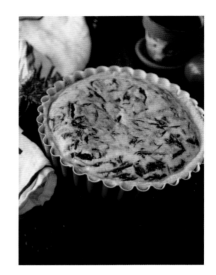

METHOD:

1. Measure out flour in a large bowl.

2. With a hand grater, grate butter into flour. Once completed, cut in butter quickly until flour mixture is coarse.

3. Add egg, water, and vinegar. Mix until just combined. Do not over mix. Do not add more liquid.

4. Toss out onto a lightly floured surface and knead until completely combined. Pie crust will be a bit crumbly. Do not over knead; only knead until completely combined.

5. Divide into two dough balls, flatten into discs, and freeze until ready to use (or put in the refrigerator for 10 minutes before rolling if you want to use it immediately).

6. When ready to use, flour surface and roll out pie crust to desired thickness, or about ¼ inch.

FOR THE QUICHE:

3 tbsp butter (or bacon grease)

2 large handfuls spinach

7 fresh eggs

2 cups heavy cream

½ tbsp thyme

½ tbsp parsley

1½ tbsp chives

salt and pepper, to taste (optional)

5 ounces fresh goat cheese

1 premade pie crust

METHOD:

1. In a skillet, melt butter and wilt spinach. Set aside to cool.

2. In a large bowl, beat together eggs and heavy cream until a bit fluffy. Add in thyme, parsley, and chives; mix well. Season with salt and pepper if desired.

3. Add cooled spinach into egg mixture and combine well. Crumble in goat cheese, leaving a little left over to garnish on top.

4. Pour mixture into pie crust that has been prepared in a tart pan or pie pan. Add remaining cheese to the top of the quiche.

5. Bake in a preheated oven at 400°F for 45–60 minutes or until the center of the quiche isn't jiggly.

6. Allow to cool for 10 minutes before cutting and serving. Serve warm.

Chicken Stock

Homemade chicken stock, also known as bone broth, is a necessity on any homestead. It can help heal a leaky gut, improve joint health by increasing collagen, boost the immune system, and even help combat food intolerances and allergies. It's so popular and necessary that it's getting a small little section all its own. If you're not making this on a regular basis, *what in the world is wrong with you?*

The health benefits of chicken stock are incredible for the human body, and this is one of the best ways to incorporate herbs into your diet so you can eat your medicine! All chicken stock begins with the same base—bones, water, vegetables, herbs. But what you decide to put in there with regard to vegetables and herbs really makes a difference. I also choose to use chicken feet in my chicken stock, as there is a lot of natural cartilage and collagen that is released that helps the body and intestinal tract heal. Here's my homegrown herbal chicken stock recipe.

leftover bones of roasted chicken carcass, picked mostly clean

chicken feet, cleaned and peeled (optional)

2 carrots, peeled and roughly chopped

1 onion, peeled and roughly chopped

2 celery stalks, cleaned and roughly chopped

1 bay leaf

4 cloves garlic

6 sprigs thyme, fresh

1 sprig rosemary, fresh

5 sprigs parsley, fresh

water to cover

METHOD:

1. Add carcass, feet (if using), vegetables, and herbs to a large stock pot. Cover with water and put lid on.

2. Bring to a boil, then bring temperature down to a low simmer for 6–8 hours.

3. Strain liquid into jars and store bone broth in the refrigerator for up to three days, use immediately in soups, or drink plain. You can also freeze or pressure can your bone broth for later use and longer storage.

Waste not, want not

Toss out the leftover bones and herbs to your farm animals. The chickens and pigs especially love them, though your chickens will appreciate them more once they cook down longer. You can also make this recipe in your crockpot and allow it to cook on a low setting all day long. Eventually, your bones will be mushy, and they can even be soft enough to feed to your dogs and other livestock.

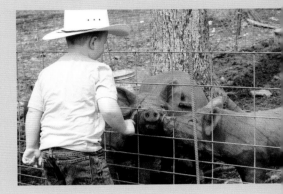

Rustic Chicken Noodle Soup

Now that you have your chicken stock, use it to make good old-fashioned chicken noodle soup! This is my make-and-take recipe for other farm families who are dealing with sickness or loss, or who are celebrating the birth of a new baby. Also, it's just fabulous on a cold winter day for your very own family! The nutrients from the bone broth and the additional herbs that are added make this a true, good-for-the-body soup for those with ailments. Feel free to add whatever you wish. Oftentimes, I'll add diced potatoes and celery as well.

2 tbsp butter

4 carrots, sliced or diced

½ onion, diced

2 cloves garlic, minced

chicken bone broth (3–4 quarts)

1 tbsp thyme, dried (or 5 fresh sprigs)

2 bay leaves

salt and pepper

4–5 chicken breasts, uncooked

2–3 cups egg noodles

METHOD:

1. In a large Dutch oven or stew pot, add butter, carrots, onions, and garlic. Cook until they begin to soften and become translucent.

2. Add chicken bone broth, thyme, bay leaves, chicken breasts, and salt and pepper. Simmer on medium low heat for 1 hour, making sure that it is at a full simmer. Simmering the soup for this long draws out the natural beta-carotene in the carrots and gives you a rich, dark, red/yellow broth in the soup. It also infuses your raw chicken with the broth and herb flavors.

3. Add 2–3 cups of egg noodles and cook for an additional 5–7 minutes, or until noodles are soft.

4. Serve hot or pour into half-gallon mason jars and store in the fridge for up to five days. You can also can the soup in a pressure canner for longer storage.

Fermented Dill and Turmeric Pickles

8 cups water

2½ tbsp pink Himalayan sea salt

pickling cucumbers (enough to fill your crock but leave headspace)

2 garlic cloves

2 tbsp dried dill, or a bunch of fresh dill (chopped)

1 tbsp each: coriander, mustard seed, and peppercorns

1 bay leaf

1 tbsp turmeric, chopped and peeled

Why do I use pink Himalayan salt?

In most of my recipes I often use pink Himalayan sea salt. It's more than just a salt; it's a nutrient-rich product full of minerals and trace elements such as calcium, potassium, copper, iron, and magnesium. It is also known as the cleanest salt on the planet. Many people still use regular table salt, and that works just as well.

METHOD:

1. Bring water to a boil in a saucepan, add salt and boil until combined. Let cool for 5 minutes.

2. Place your cucumbers in your crock, leaving enough headspace for liquid to fill in.

3. Add remaining dry ingredients and turmeric to the crock, and then pour salt brine over cucumbers until they are completely submerged.

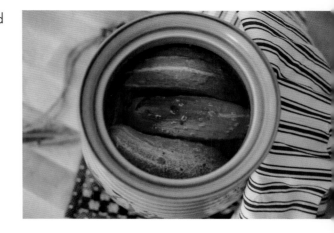

4. If your cucumbers begin to float, add a fermentation weight or heavy bowl to the top. Cover the top of your crock with a secured towel and rubber band or string.

5. Allow to ferment on your countertop for at least seven days. They will smell delightful! When finished, place into cans and refrigerate to slow the fermentation process, or keep them in a cool place in your pantry or root cellar (in the crock or in new jars), and they will continue to ferment until you're ready to eat them.

Fermented Dilly Beans

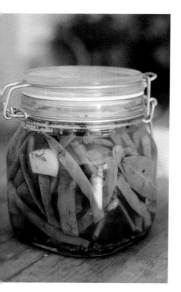

Dilly beans are my absolute favorite fermenting vegetable. I even freeze some of our green bean harvest so that I can make dilly beans all year long. They are truly a delicious treat for everyone in the family!

This recipe is very similar to the dill pickle recipe, but the taste is quite different.

8 cups water

2½ tbsp pink Himalayan salt

Green beans, washed and trimmed (enough to fill a mason jar)

2 garlic cloves

2 tbsp dried dill, or a bunch of fresh dill (chopped)

½ tbsp each: coriander, mustard seed, and peppercorns

1 bay leaf

Where to store

While root cellar and pantry storage can be beneficial with ferments, there is some concern that they could become contaminated. This is why I prefer to cap my ferments tightly and place them in the fridge once they have reached the desired taste.

METHOD:

1. Bring water to a boil in a saucepan, add salt and boil until combined. Let cool for 5 minutes.

2. Place your green beans in a mason jar or container of choice, leaving enough headspace for liquid to fill in.

3. Add remaining dry ingredients into the container, and then pour salt brine over the green beans until they are completely submerged.

4. If your beans begin to float, add a fermentation weight or heavy bowl to the top. Cover the top of your container with a secured towel and rubber band or string.

5. Allow to ferment on your counter top for 4–6 days. They will quickly smell delightful, and beans don't need as much time to ferment as some other vegetables (like cucumbers). When finished, refrigerate the beans (capped tightly) to slow the fermentation process, or keep them in a cool place in your pantry or root cellar (in the container or in new jars), and they will continue to ferment (though slowly, in a cool place) until you're ready to eat them.

Thyme Biscuits

Thyme is my favorite herb. Biscuits are my favorite bread. You see what I did here? Yes, you want these to be on your dinner table—or better yet, your holiday table. These biscuits pair exquisitely well with old country, salty, yummy ham.

The only issue with making biscuits? You really have to *feel* your way into the perfect biscuit dough. People often have such a hard time making biscuits because they don't understand the technique. I never use a recipe for biscuits, but I've tried to put this one together for you. And I'll try to convey the technique in an easy-to-understand way.

4 cups all-purpose flour, unbleached

2½ tsp baking powder

1 tbsp thyme, dried

½ lb butter, cold

1–2 cups milk

additional butter for pan

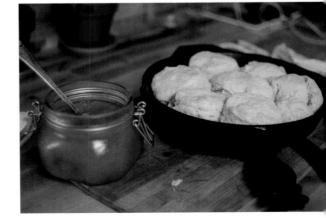

METHOD:

1. Preheat oven to 375°F.

2. Add flour, baking powder, and thyme to a large bowl. Mix well.

3. With a hand grater, grate the cold butter into your flour mixture, working quickly so that the butter doesn't melt too much. Coat the butter well with the flour mixture until your mixture is coarse.

4. Add 1 cup of milk. Mix well. Add additional milk if necessary in $1/2$-cup increments. The dough should be handled as little as possible. You want it to be very dense and a bit crumbly but not sticky.

5. Once mixed, turn dough out onto a floured surface. Fold the dough over onto itself about ten times. The folding technique will cause your dough to rise higher and create a fluffier, layered biscuit.

6. Pat dough flat, about $1–1^1/_2$ inch in thickness, and cut into biscuit shapes with a round cookie cutter or mason jar. Place biscuits, with sides touching, in a buttered cast-iron skillet. Make sure the sides are touching something at all times, as this causes the biscuits to rise better as well.

7. Bake until tops of biscuits begin to turn golden (about 20–30 minutes). Remove from oven and allow to cool for about 5 minutes. They will be extremely hot.

8. Serve warm with butter or honey. Or allow to cool and use for ham biscuits.

Easy Herb Pesto

Pesto isn't something I'm necessarily wild about in its plain form. I know, don't stone me. But it is something that I enjoy cooking with. This is a great way to use up the extra basil you have in your garden. Use it on or in breads, on pasta, in salads, and more! You can even freeze it in ice cube trays for later use.

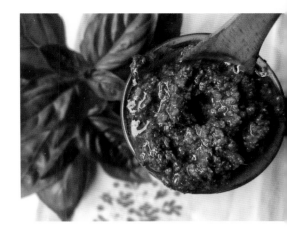

3–4 cups fresh basil

2 cloves garlic

1 tsp lemon zest

1½ tsp lemon juice

¼ cup toasted pine nuts

½ cup grated parmesan cheese

½ cup olive oil

METHOD:

1. Add all ingredients, except olive oil, to a food processor. Pulse until ingredients are minced.

2. Slowly drizzle in olive oil, with processor on, until it emulsifies and combines with all of the ingredients. Your pesto should be creamy and well combined.

3. Store in your refrigerator in a container until ready to use, or freeze in ice cube trays for later use. It will last 5–7 days in the fridge, and up to eight months in the freezer.

Herb Salad Dressing

Have fun with this creamy herb salad dressing! It's a great alternative to the store-bought ranch version.

3 tbsp chives, thinly chopped

½ cup fresh basil, thinly chopped

1 heaping tbsp fresh dill

½ tbsp garlic powder

1 tbsp Dijon mustard

1 tsp salt

1 tsp black pepper

1 tbsp olive oil

juice of 1 lemon

½ cup Greek yogurt

½ cup whipping cream

METHOD:

1. Add all ingredients, except yogurt and whipping cream, to a food processor. Combine for 20 seconds or until smooth.

2. Add yogurt and whipping cream and combine until mixture is silky smooth. Cover and allow to set in the refrigerator for 1 hour or overnight.

3. Use on salads or as a dipping sauce!

Vinaigrette combos

Parsley, chives, cilantro, and dill

Garlic, basil, and oregano

Parsley, basil, oregano, lemon juice, and parmesan cheese

Lemon juice, mint, sundried tomatoes, and basil

Parmesan cheese, basil, garlic, and onion

Herb Vinaigrette

Herb vinaigrettes are so easy to make. Once you learn, your combinations will be endless. You'll start by using a 1-pint mason jar as your mixing tool. Here's what you'll need:

2–3 tbsp raw honey

½ cup apple cider vinegar

½ cup oil (olive oil or infused olive oil)

¼ cup fresh herbs (or 2–3 tbsp dried herbs)

METHOD:

Pour all ingredients into the mason jar. Shake vigorously. Pour onto your salad!

Lemon-Lavender Pound Cake

My grandma used to make the best pound cake ever. She would even make her regular cakes more like pound cakes because she enjoyed eating them plain without icing. My love for cake probably stems from her, but it also spoiled me—as an adult, I just don't like fluffy, light cakes. Give me the dense, thick pound cakes, and you'll be my best friend forever. Pound cakes aren't for sissies . . . they're for farmers. Enjoy the simplicity of this old-fashioned lemon pound cake, with a hint of lavender and a drizzle of sweetness.

1 cup salted butter, softened

1½ cups sugar (or raw evaporated cane juice)

2 tsp lemon zest, finely grated

juice of ½ a lemon

1 tbsp vanilla extract

5 eggs

2 cups unbleached flour

1–2 tsp lavender buds

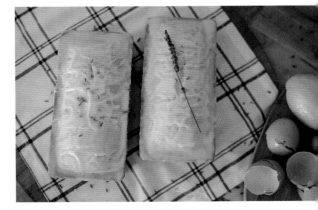

METHOD:

1. Preheat the oven to 325°F.

2. Flour two small loaf pans or one bundt pan. Set aside.

3. In a large bowl, cream butter and sugar. Beat in lemon zest, lemon juice, vanilla extract, and eggs. Combine well, then add 1–2 tsp of lavender buds and mix well.

4. Fold in flour in small batches until it's all well combined. Do not over mix.

5. Pour batter into loaf pans or bundt pan. Bake for 45–55 minutes, or until a knife or skewer comes out clean when poked. If the cake begins to brown too quickly, cover with foil.

6. Allow cake to cool in pan for about 10 minutes, then remove and continue cooling on a wire rack until cooled completely.

FOR THE DRIZZLE:

2 cups powdered sugar

4–5 tsp milk

1 tsp vanilla

¼ tsp lemon zest

METHOD:

Combine all ingredients until a thick but liquid mixture comes together. Drizzle over warm loaf so that it begins to soak into the cake.

Chocolate Peppermint Pudding

This pudding is my favorite thing to snack on during the holidays. The peppermint essential oil brings a hint of wintertime to the mix, and the pudding itself is rich and decadent. Of course, it's not that healthy for my thighs and hips, but hey, I like to live a little! We all need a treat every now and then. The other downside? This pudding cooks quickly, so you'll need to plan on babysitting it the entire time. But it is *so* worth it.

1 cup sugar (or evaporated cane juice)

¼ cup cornstarch

3 cups fresh whole milk (raw milk is amazing!)

4 whole egg yolks, beaten

5 ounces bittersweet chocolate, finely chopped (or chips)

2 tsp vanilla extract

3 tbsp salted butter

3–4 drops peppermint essential oil (to your taste!)

METHOD:

1. In a large saucepan, combine sugar and cornstarch. Slowly add milk and beaten egg yolks and combine well.

2. Turn the saucepan on medium heat until the mixture is right below the boiling point. **Do not boil.** This process will happen in about 5–7 minutes. You'll really need to babysit this part of the process.

3. When the mixture begins to bubble, allow it to reach a pudding-like consistency, then immediately remove from heat. Add in the chocolate, vanilla, and butter. Add in 3–4 drops of peppermint, less or more to your taste. Stir until combined.

4. Eat warm or allow to cool in a container in the fridge. I prefer mine warm, but that's just me!

Note: If you don't like peppermint essential oil, you can substitute with peppermint leaves by infusing them in warm milk until they release their volatile oils.

Honey Ginger Switchel

I'll admit, I didn't grow up with *Little House on the Prairie*. I know, right? Shocker. I feel like I've been deprived of a good childhood. However, I've fallen in love with it as an adult. This ginger switchel is mentioned in one of the books by Laura Ingalls Wilder, where she talks about her mama making ginger-water when the boys were out working. She said that plain, ice cold water would upset their stomachs, but this ginger water wouldn't. She added sugar, vinegar, and ginger to warm their stomachs so that they could drink the water and their bodies could absorb the water better.

There's actually something to be said for this. I think she absolutely knew what she was doing. Enjoy this switchel on a hot summer day in the field or just as a delightful ginger drink.

8 cups of cold distilled water

3 tbsp raw apple cider vinegar

5 tbsp raw honey

4-inch piece grated ginger, cleaned and peeled first

juice from ½ a lemon (optional)

METHOD:

1. Mix/shake all ingredients together in a large mason jar. Allow to set for a few minutes.

2. Drink the switchel straight from the jar, or you can pour the switchel through a strainer into individual cups after it has set in the refrigerator for 24 hours if you prefer to make it in advance and don't want to drink the grated ginger pieces.

Chai Tea Latte

This warming tea is the perfect cup to have on hand when you're a mama. I mean, really, it's just the best thing—whether it's spring or fall. Turn the tea into a latte, and it's pure heaven.

You'll need to begin with whole spices and grind them down yourself for the most potent tea. But it's okay if you've already ground your herbs and are making the mix in advance, which is what we're doing with this recipe.

1 tbsp ground black pepper

2 tbsp ground ginger

2 tsp ground allspice

2 tbsp ground cardamom

1½ tbsp ground cinnamon

1 tsp ground cloves

1 tsp grated nutmeg

3 star anise pods, whole

In a container, mix together all spices. Do not grind up the star anise pods, as they add flavor to the mix as it sets over time.

When you're ready to make your tea (by the cupful)—

green tea, black tea, or rooibos tea

½ –2 tsp chai mix

orange zest (optional)

½ tsp vanilla extract

1 tbsp raw honey or sweetener of choice (if using whipped cream, you can omit sweetener)

dash of cream (optional)

homemade whipped cream (optional)

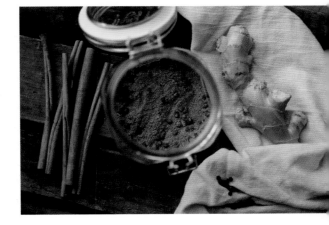

METHOD:

1. Steep tea of choice in a cup.

2. Add ½-2 teaspoons of chai mix to cup, combine well. This will be completely made to your taste and liking. You can strain the herbs from the tea once it finishes steeping or drink it as is. The herbs will naturally fall to the bottom of the cup.

3. Sprinkle in a bit of orange zest if you like, along with vanilla extract, your sweetener, and cream. Top with homemade whipped cream, if desired. (Of course you desire—it makes it ten times better!)

Respiratory Marshmallow Hot Cocoa

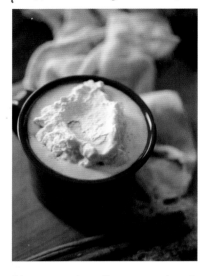

Wintertime often brings with it inflamed sore throats and respiratory tract problems. There's nothing quite like coming inside to a hot cup of cocoa, but marshmallow root makes it that much better. This herb will help reduce coughing, sore throat, and inflammation in the respiratory tract and is even safe for the little helping hands. Using raw milk in this recipe will further decrease inflammation and soothe the respiratory tract, and the marshmallow brings a cinnamon flavor to the drink. This recipe makes enough for 8 cups of hot chocolate.

³/₄ oz marshmallow root, dried

9 cups milk (raw is best!)

½ cup sugar

¼ cup cocoa powder (good quality)

1 tsp vanilla extract

METHOD:

1. In a saucepan, heat up milk and marshmallow root. Allow to infuse for 30 minutes without bringing to a boil but still very hot. Once complete, strain out marshmallow root (if you did not use a tea bag or tea infuser) and return milk to hot saucepan.

2. Add sugar, melt, and combine completely.

3. Add cocoa powder and stir until completely combined.

4. Add vanilla extract and combine well.

5. Serve warm with homemade whipped cream or marshmallows . . . the big fluffy kind.

It's exciting to see herbs used throughout every part of our home. From herbal medicine to eating herbs at the dinner table, herbs are so versatile and can be incorporated into so many aspects of our lives.

In the next chapter, I'll walk you right out to the backyard (and barnyard) and show you how you can incorporate herbs around your outbuildings to help with pests, maintain healthy pets and livestock, and clean with natural herbal cleaners and sprays.

Let's go!

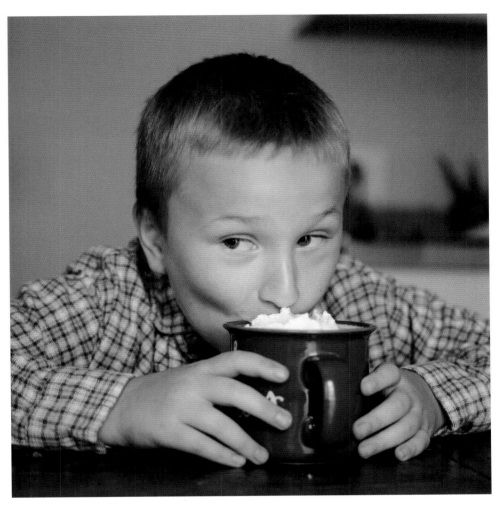

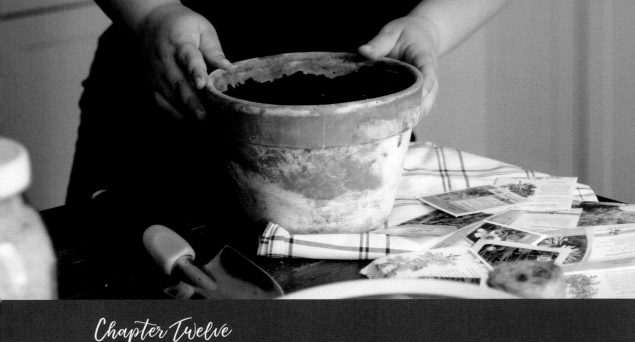

Chapter Twelve

HERBS FOR THE HOME AND BARN

The barn. Where do I begin? Let's just remember to be thankful for how good the manure from our livestock is for our gardens, because that's about all manure is good for. I mean, really, don't you just love the smell of fresh manure in the morning? Even more lovely is the cleaning out of the barn. Oh yes, that's some fresh manure goodness right there. Mmm mmmm.

After a good barn cleaning, we trek our messes into the house. *Gosh, what a pigsty.* There are dishes scattered about. There's a dirt ring around the bathtub, laundry to be put away, and a nice glob of mud on the floor.

Isn't farm life just glorious?

You might be inclined to reach for the bottle of cleaner and spray everything down. But wait, have you thought about what's in that cleaner you're using? I mean, we're homesteaders, right? We are homesteading because we want to live a natural lifestyle, right?

Darn it, what am I doing with this chemical in my hand?!

Look around you. Every single cleaner you use, every single detergent or air freshener, has some type of chemical in it, even some of your "natural" ones. Or worse, they have ingredients that you can't even pronounce. Without realizing it, many of the household and barn products that we use to keep our environment sanitary and smelling fresh can have long-term detriments to our health, the health of our livestock, and the natural world in general.

Fortunately, almost everything you use on a regular basis in your home and around your barn has an easy-to-make herbal alternative. You can produce your own air fresheners, window cleaners, wood floor polishes, and more. And this will cost you less than all the chemical stuff, and even the cleaners that are labeled "all natural," which is often an excuse for manufacturers to raise the price!

Let's break it down by chore and building. Many of the cleaners and herbal products that you make can be used on just about all surfaces and for multiple uses—kind of a "one size fits all."

Keep in mind that you should always try to use glass spray bottles. And most created products should be kept in a temperature-controlled area rather than in a hot area or in direct sunlight. Also, use up each mixture within six months.

Why glass bottles?

While you most certainly can use plastic bottles to hold your herbal preparations, it's best to use glass bottles, as plastic can leach into the product, and eventually the oils and vinegar (or vodka) can begin to break down the plastic. Plus, glass bottles are just prettier!

ALL-PURPOSE HOME HERBAL CLEANER

This is my favorite product, ever. I'm going to give you two different options to clean with—one with essential oils and one with herbs. I find that I tend more toward the essential oil recipe, because it's quick and easy to make. But there are times I do really enjoy the cleaning power of the herb-infused cleaner, especially when I need to deep clean.

Cleaner with Essential Oils

7 oz white vinegar

7 oz distilled water

30 drops lemon essential oil

10 drops tea tree essential oil

METHOD:

1. Fill a 16-ounce amber glass spray bottle halfway with white vinegar and fill the remaining half with distilled water, leaving a 2-inch headspace before you get to the cap part of the bottle.

2. Add your essential oils. Cap and shake well.

3. Before each use, shake your bottle, and continue to shake it periodically while using it. This ensures that your oils stay mixed together.

Note: The lemon oil in this recipe helps degrease and leaves behind a fresh scent. The tea tree oil in the recipe is naturally antiseptic and cleans up any lingering bacteria. Vinegar is a natural sanitizer, and is basically bleach's herbal alternative. However, the real power is not in the vinegar itself, but when it dries. Therefore, when cleaning with vinegar, don't wipe the vinegar away with a dry rag. Allow it to evaporate on its own.

Cleaner with Herbs

thyme, sage, peppermint (handfuls, bruised with a mortar and pestle)

1 lemon, sliced

white vinegar

witch hazel

distilled water

METHOD:

1. In a large glass jar (quart and half-gallon sizes work well), add handfuls of your favorite herbs. I include thyme, sage, and peppermint, with a major emphasis on peppermint. The ratio will be roughly 1 part herbs to 3 parts liquid (vinegar).

2. Add sliced lemon, squeezing the slices as you add them.

3. Add 3 parts white vinegar to the jar, enough to cover the herbs and lemon, just enough so they don't poke above the vinegar.

4. Cap tightly and allow to sit on the counter or in the pantry, out of direct sunlight, for two weeks. Shake each day.

5. Once your mixture is finished extracting, strain the liquid into a new jar, cap, and keep in the refrigerator until you're ready to use it.

6. When ready to make a bottle of your cleaning solution, pour your mixture into half of a 16-ounce glass spray bottle. Fill the remaining part of the bottle with 1 part water and 1 part witch hazel. Shake before each use.

Note: This solution, once mixed with your water and witch hazel, can be kept in your cleaning closet. However, keep whatever liquid hasn't been mixed in your refrigerator to extend its shelf life.

Herbal Goop Gone

The first time I made this recipe, I used it on wallpaper in my kitchen that was giving me a fit while I was trying to remove it. I bought the chemical stuff (silly me!). It didn't work. So, I made up a bottle of this "goop gone" and guess what, the goop is gone, y'all! That nasty floral wallpaper came right off after I sprayed it. You'll note that the recipe calls for 20 drops of lemon essential oil, but this will depend on your bottle size. Making a small batch? Use 10 drops. For larger batches, use the 20 drops. Use this on anything sticky that needs to be removed naturally.

water

1 tbsp of natural dish liquid

20 drops lemon essential oil

5 drops thyme essential oil

METHOD:

Fill a 16-ounce spray bottle a little less than three-quarters of the way with water. Add dish liquid and essential oils. Shake well.

Essential Oil Floor Cleaner

I'm not sure I'll ever go back to commercial floor cleaner. I even use this mixture on my wood floors, and it has always done very well for me. The dish liquid in this recipe is optional. Many times I don't use it unless I need extra-strength cleaning. You do not need to rinse the floor with clean water if you use dish liquid, as you are using a minimal amount. For an exceptionally soiled floor, you should probably go over it twice with your mop.

hot tap water

6 drops lavender essential oil

6 drops lemongrass essential oil

4 drops eucalyptus essential oil

¼ cup white vinegar

1 tbsp natural liquid soap (optional)

METHOD:

1. Fill mop bucket up with hot tap water, adding essential oils, vinegar, and soap to the bucket as it fills.

2. Mop floors thoroughly. Dispose of liquid when finished.

Four Thieves Plague Cleaner

This cleaner sounds really creepy, doesn't it? The folklore behind it gives it its name. Long story short, during one of the plagues, a family began robbing grave sites of the people who died. Miraculously, they never ended up getting the plague themselves. But they were eventually arrested. When asked what their secret was to staying healthy, they revealed it in exchange for their freedom. Turns out, they would cover their bodies with a blend of peppermint, lavender, rosemary, and sage essential oils. They would also cleanse the items they stole with this blend. Over the centuries, we've begun to perfect the blend by adding more oils of our own. Does this cleaner get rid of sickness and plagues? No idea. But I can confidently tell you that it is naturally antiseptic, antibacterial, and antiviral.

2 cups white vinegar

20 drops rosemary essential oil

20 drops sage essential oil

20 drops peppermint essential oil

25 drops lemon essential oil

15 drops eucalyptus essential oil

2 smashed garlic cloves

METHOD:

In a 16-ounce glass spray bottle, combine all ingredients and shake well. You can use immediately, or for better results, allow it to set for 24–48 hours so the garlic has time to extract. Use this spray on door handles, toilet seats, phones, and other surfaces that need to be sanitized during times of illness. It's also just a great cleaner for all-purpose cleaning. I really enjoy using this in the barn as well. Use within one year of making.

Homemade Air Freshener

You'll never have to buy air freshener again. You can switch up the essential oils in this recipe for any season or aroma. In the fall, I often like to use clove, cedarwood, and cinnamon. And during the holidays, Douglas fir, peppermint, and white fir essential oils are my favorites. Just make sure that you shake the bottle before each use. The witch hazel acts as a binding agent with the oils and water.

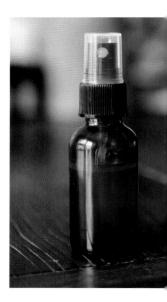

water

witch hazel

4 drops lemongrass essential oil

4 drops grapefruit essential oil

2 drops sage essential oil

METHOD:

1. Fill a 1-ounce glass spray bottle a little over halfway with water.

2. Add witch hazel to the remaining space in the bottle, leaving room for essential oils.

3. Add essential oils and shake well.

4. Shake well before each use to make sure the mixture is well combined.

My favorite air fresheners

Pumpkin Spice: 3 drops clove • 2 drops cassia • 2 drops ginger • 1 drop cardamom

Winter Wonderland: 4 drops Siberian fir • 2 drops cinnamon • 2 drops Douglas fir • 1 drop clove • 1 drop tangerine

Into the Woods: 3 drops bergamot • 3 drops vetiver • 2 drops cedarwood

Lemon Clean: 4 drops lemongrass • 2 drops tangerine

Relax and Uplift: 3 drops lime • 2 drops lavender • 2 drops myrrh • 1 drop cedarwood

Natural Window and Glass Cleaner

2 cups white vinegar

½ cup distilled water

10 drops wild orange essential oil (or any citrus oil)

5 drops peppermint essential oil

METHOD:

1. Combine all ingredients in a spray bottle.

2. Shake before each use. Spray on windows or glass as you would with any other glass cleaner and then wipe clean.

Note: You can also use this same recipe to clean your glass stovetop, microwave, and other kitchen appliances.

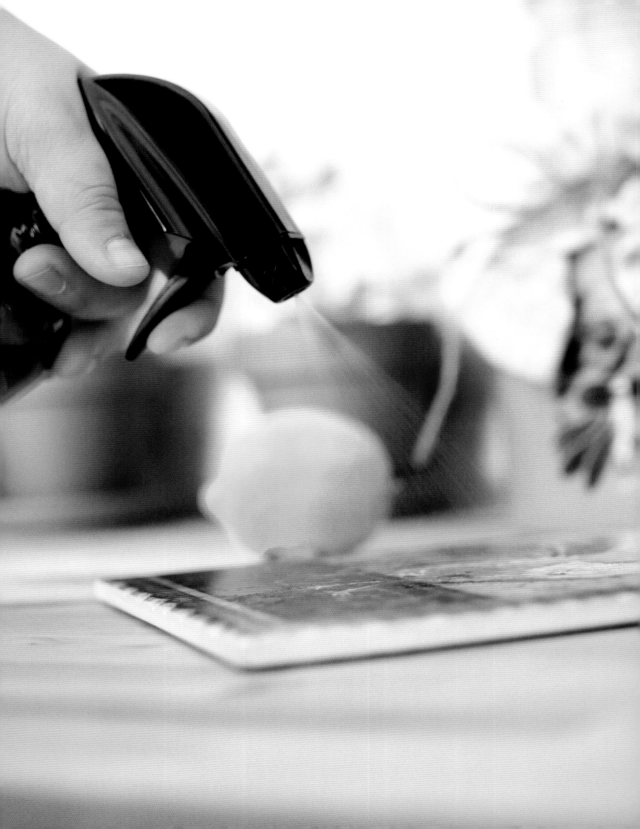

Wool Dryer Balls with Essential Oils (Dryer Sheet Alternative)

Dryer sheets are a huge issue in modern society; the chemicals contained in some of them emit VOCs (volatile organic compounds) that are known to be toxic to people after sustained exposure, and may even be linked to diseases such as Alzheimer's and cancer. So why are we still using them in our homes? Dryer balls are a natural alternative to dryer sheets, and they help your clothes dry faster as well. Simply add 6 drops of essential oil onto each of your dryer balls (4–6 balls) and use them as you would dryer sheets. That's it!

Lemon and Tea Tree Dusting Spray

Dusting. It's my least favorite chore to do. Why? Because I always forget about it. I mean, who really thinks about dusting until there's an inch of dust on the shelves? Maybe more people than I realize. Either way, this recipe is equally as good as that nasty chemical-filled spray you can buy from the store!

distilled water

white vinegar

½ cup olive oil

15 drops lemon essential oil

8 drops tea tree essential oil

5 drops cedarwood essential oil (optional)

METHOD:

1. Fill a 16-ounce spray bottle, with 1 part distilled water and 1 part vinegar.

2. Add ½ cup olive oil and essential oils. Shake to combine well.

3. Shake before each use, and use as you would any regular dusting spray.

The importance of distilled water

You may notice that many of these recipes call for distilled water instead of tap water, and there's a good reason why. If your water is chemically treated, the chemicals will literally kill the benefits of the herbs and essential oils in your household cleaning products. If you're on well water, salt and minerals can have a similar effect on herbs and oils. For this reason, I always suggest distilled water to avoid any chemicals, impurities, and excessive salts and minerals.

HERBS AROUND THE BARNYARD

One morning, I tied a string to a bundle of herbs—peppermint, thyme, and sage, to be exact—and walked down to the chicken coop. I had planned on giving the herbs to one of our mama rabbits that had just finished weaning, but as I looked

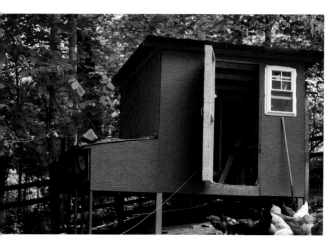

around my chicken coop, I realized that the bundle should be used for something else. My coop was looking a little dingy and needed a good freshening up, and the chickens were in need of a pick-me-up on that autumn day while in the middle of their yearly molt. Chickens molt their feathers every single year and trade them in for fresh new feathers. During this time, they are extremely tired, less likely to forage, and could use a few immune-boosting treats. I decided then and there to hang the bundle about a foot from the coop floor to serve as a freshener and a way for the chickens to get some herbs in their diet.

My newfound love for herbalism was now extending past my own household into the barnyard. I realized I could do so much more with herbs around the coop, in the hutches, the nesting boxes, the waterers, and more. I could even plant herbs around my outbuildings to deter pests! Who would've thought it?

HERBS TO DETER PESTS AROUND OUTBUILDINGS

More often than not, I find myself drawn to picking a bouquet of herbs rather than flowers, (although, I can't help throwing in a few zinnias here and there). Not only are herbs fragrant and beautiful planted around the homestead, they also provide real benefits to you and your farm animals. You'll always have rodents and insects lurking around, but here are a few herbs that are pretty and can also help keep those pests in check:

Peppermint: deters ants, spiders, small rodents, aphids, flea beetles, cabbage pests, and helps deter mosquitoes. It is also an herb that you can plant once and then it spreads like wildfire.

Lemon Balm: deters mosquitoes and other insects, attracts butterflies and bees. Rub areas down with lemon balm, or plant or hang bundles of it in and around outbuildings.

Basil: deters flies and mosquitoes.

Calendula: deters rats and small rodents.

Wormwood: deters mice, rats, and small rodents.

Cayenne: deters rats, small rodents, beetles, and other insects. Sprinkle powdered cayenne on the floor of your coop and barn as well to get rid of unwanted pests and bugs.

HERB BUNDLES

My favorite thing to do with herbs around the barnyard is to hang them in bundles—whether it's in the coop, a barn, or a rabbit hutch. Herb bundles bring so much more benefit than we realize. They can be fragrant and aromatic health enhancers for our animals and ourselves. Our livestock rub up against them and get the scent on them, which can help deter pests.. Our chickens peck at the

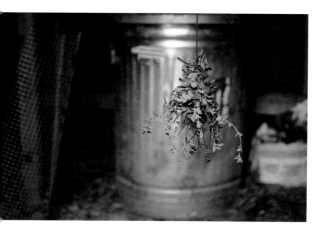

bundles and get their daily intake of herbs that help keep them healthy and thriving. They can also be boredom busters during rainy or snowy days.

Most of the herbs included in the following recipes work well for all livestock. When in doubt, consult a professional or do a little research, as each herb bundle can have a different effect on animals. The herb bundles can be as small or as large as you wish, but I would suggest the size of a bouquet of flowers (think a dozen roses). If you need more bundles for more animals, instead of making a larger bundle, just make multiple smaller bundles and spread them throughout the area. Here are my favorites.

New Mama Herb Bundle

This bundle includes herbs that help encourage lactation and calmness in a new barnyard mother. Be careful to wear gloves while preparing the bundle if you are sensitive to stinging nettle.

Red Raspberry Leaf	Comfrey
Stinging Nettle	Lavender
Fennel	

Going Dry Herb Bundle

This is the bundle I use most for mamas that are currently weaning or are just post-weaning. These herbs encourage the drying up of milk and help make it less stressful on mama.

Sage	Thyme	Peppermint

General Health Herb Bundle

Want to give your livestock an extra boost in their diet? This herb bundle is the way to go. Now, if you're hanging this bundle in a barn, I'm pretty sure the milk cow is going to eat it all in one munch. But if you're feeding it to smaller livestock, like ducks, chickens, and rabbits, it will last a lot longer. Instead of the bundle, you can also add these herbs to the diet of your larger livestock. We'll go over that more in another chapter.

Oregano

Thyme

Peppermint

Garlic (with scapes)

Onion (with scapes)

Aromatic Herb Bundle

Just looking to spruce up the outbuildings with beautiful and aromatic herb bundles? This is the one for you. I make this almost weekly in the summer months when fresh herbs are growing, and it never disappoints! Dry out these herbs in large bundles in the summer and store them in an airtight container for winter use.

Lavender

Sage

Oregano

Peppermint/Spearmint

Rosemary

Lemon Balm

ESSENTIAL OIL RAGS

After herb bundles, my second favorite thing is to make essential oil rags. I often use these when I need to aromatically soothe or help keep pests away from my livestock. You simply sprinkle drops of essential oils on rag strips and hang them strategically to suit you and your livestock's needs. Keep in mind that these rags are used in open rather than confined spaces. If using in extra-small hutches or coops, cut each recipe in half.

You could use an electric essential oil diffuser in your coop or barn, but I find that the rags are more effective and cover a larger area. You also don't have to fear your livestock knocking them over.

Use this first recipe as a basis for all your other rag recipes.

Basic Essential Oil Rag Strips

  5 strips of old rags

  10–20 drops of essential oils (total)

Add essential oils to rag strips (10–20 drops total, not per rag). These 5 strips will fill up an 8x8-foot coop with its aroma. If you have a larger space, you'll need to make more rag strips and space them strategically throughout the building.

Good-bye Fly Essential Oil Rag Strips

Hang in your coop or outbuilding to deter flies and other unwanted flying pests. Because, who has time to deal with flies!? These rags will last several days. Yes, we actually use these and they certainly do work. You can use the same rags over again. Just wash them out thoroughly under the hose, set in the sun to dry, and start all over again.

  7 drops tea tree essential oil

  6 drops oregano essential oil

  4 drops lemon balm essential oil

Calming Essential Oil Rag Strips

I really enjoy using these rags during times when my livestock has been stressed. This might be after a predator attack, when a mama is in labor, or in the winter months when they are cooped up inside because of the snow. Plus, it just makes everything smell good!

  5 drops lavender essential oil

  4 drops chamomile essential oil

  4 drops rose essential oil

Respiratory Essential Oil Rag Strips

This works especially well for chickens when their respiratory tracts are inflamed due to dust, allergens, or respiratory distress. These oils not only help open up the airways but also help heal and soothe the lining of the respiratory tract through aromatics. These rag strips work well for all livestock.

> 5 drops peppermint essential oil
>
> 4 drops eucalyptus (*E. radiata*) essential oil
>
> 4 drops basil essential oil
>
> 3 drops tea tree essential oil

HERBAL BARNYARD PRODUCTS

Whether it's fly spray, coop cleaner, or black drawing salve, there are many herbal alternatives that are easy to make and use for the barnyard. Often, they're even more effective than chemical-based products.

One product can accomplish many different things. For example, the barn cleaner can be used anywhere as a cleaner. And the fly spray can be sprayed in your coop as well as on your cows. Black drawing salve can be used on any animal for many different things—rooster comb frostbite, open wounds, and even bumblefoot.

Barn and Coop Cleaner

This coop cleaner is effective and aggressive, and, it smells lovely! Vodka and white vinegar are natural cleaners and are used often in sterilization. Vodka, in fact, was used in hospitals and doctors' offices to sterilize surgical utensils. This barn cleaner can be used full strength in a glass spray bottle, or it can be diluted with half water and half extraction mixture. The choice is really up to you. I prefer to use mine full strength at least once a month so that it sterilizes efficiently.

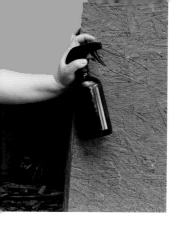

the peels from 3 oranges

1 cup mint, chopped (peppermint or spearmint)

¼ cup lavender buds

2 sprigs rosemary

1 handful sage

white vinegar (or vodka)

METHOD:

1. Combine peels and herbs in a large mason jar.

2. Cover herbs completely with white vinegar or vodka.

3. Allow to set for 2–4 weeks, then strain into a new glass jar until ready to use in a glass spray bottle.

Herbal Coop Freshener with Herbs

I make two different versions of this recipe—one with herbs and one with essential oils. I'll give you both versions. The herbal freshener is my go-to because I absolutely love the scent of vanilla in my coop. But more than that, the oregano and mint help deter flies and other unwanted pests. Simply spray the coop and other outbuildings in the morning for a nice freshening up.

the peels from 3 lemons

the peel from 1 orange

2 vanilla beans

½ cup mint, chopped (peppermint or spearmint)

½ cup oregano

½ cup sage

1 tbsp cloves

white vinegar

water

METHOD:

1. Combine peels, vanilla beans, and herbs into a large mason jar.

2. Cover herbs completely with white vinegar.

3. Allow to set for 2–4 weeks, then strain into a new glass jar until ready to use in a glass spray bottle. When ready to use, cut with water if aroma is too pungent.

Herbal Coop Freshener with Essential Oils

An essential oil freshener is much easier than waiting for an herbal freshener to extract during a two- to four-week time period. I often alternate during those time periods—a few weeks with herbs, a few weeks with essential oils. One of the most fabulous things about this freshener is that it can also be used as a cleaning spray, as all of the essential oils mentioned have cleaning and sanitizing properties. The addition of witch hazel not only combines the oils with the water to allow it to make an aromatic freshener, but it is also a natural cleaning agent.

distilled water

witch hazel

6 drops tea tree essential oil

6 drops lemongrass essential oil

8 drops oregano essential oil

2 drops clove essential oil

3 drops sage essential oil

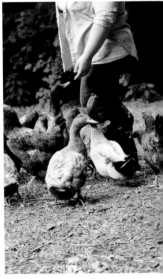

METHOD:

1. Fill a 16-ounce spray bottle a little less than three-quarters of the way with water. Then add witch hazel to nearly fill the bottle, leaving room to add essential oils.

2. Add essential oils to bottle and shake well to combine. Shake before each use. Store in a temperature-controlled area for up to six months.

Powerhouse Natural Fly Spray

There's nothing worse than flies or mosquitoes all over your family milk cow in the hot summer months while you're milking. Not only is it frustrating to you, but it's frustrating to your livestock as well. Making up a jug of this fly spray will certainly help ease everyone's frustrations. I do suggest making a large jug and then portioning it out into smaller spray bottles as you need it. Try to use up the entire jug within 1–2 weeks because after a week, the oils start to deteriorate.

Also, don't waste your time using raw apple cider vinegar for this. The witch hazel and essential oils alone will kill the good bacteria in the vinegar. Just shoot for the regular stuff. Alternatively, you can create a fly spray without the oils and witch hazel; just use fresh herbs boiled down into a spray, and then add the vinegar without the witch hazel or essential oils. However, it's not as potent, and requires more spraying.

2 cups apple cider vinegar

15 drops lemongrass essential oil

15 drops rosemary essential oil

15 drops basil essential oil

15 drops peppermint essential oil

15 drops cedarwood essential oil

5 drops eucalyptus essential oil

2 drops citronella essential oil (optional)

1 smashed clove of garlic

2 tbsp natural dish soap

distilled water

witch hazel or vodka

METHOD:

1. In a large jug (64-ounce or similar) combine apple cider vinegar, essential oils, garlic, and dish soap.

2. Add distilled water so that the entire mixture fills the jug a little less than three-quarters of the way full.

3. Fill remaining space in jug with witch hazel or vodka. Shake well to combine. Use within 1–2 weeks, adding the mixture to a spray bottle when ready to use. Keep jug in a temperature-controlled area so that your mixture doesn't deteriorate quickly.

There's no excuse for the barn or your bathroom to be stinky now that you have these recipes! And the best part is that you and your livestock won't mind the scents, which are not only beneficial but bring a sense of calm to your home and barnyard.

We won't stop at cleaners and fly sprays on the homestead. I'm about to show you another way to use herbs on your homestead, farm, or in your backyard. It's been used all over the world and is beneficial to every animal and human that comes into contact with it.

Keep it cool

I suggest keeping mixtures made with oils in a temperature-controlled environment until ready to use. While essential oils are powerful, they can become unstable and begin to break down in extreme temperature changes and when mixed with other substances.

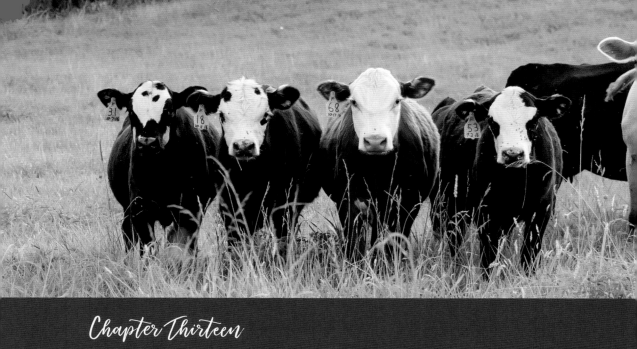

Chapter Thirteen

HERBS FOR OUR FOUR-LEGGED FRIENDS

We all love our four-legged friends, whether it's a cow or the farm dog. In this chapter we'll specifically address cows, goats, dogs, rabbits, and other four-legged animals on your homestead.

As we learn about the benefits of herbalism, we wish to be more holistic in our approach to maintaining healthy livestock and pets. Health in our animals begins with the food that we offer them. One of the best practices you can begin on your homestead is adding herbs to their feed. Of course, there are multiple different ways to do this. Let's go over a few of them.

Livestock and other animals naturally forage for wild plants if you allow them to. Typically, they'll know what they can and cannot eat. If we pasture-raise our animals and allow them to free range, we become more aware of their daily intake of food. What are they eating? Where is it coming from? Are we harvesting meat and milk from a cow that ate chemical-laden food? Are we using products from livestock that's been treated chemically for a respiratory illness? These are all questions we'll ask ourselves at some point.

What we often don't realize is just how simple it is to not only give our animals herbal supplements and treatments but to offer them a diet that helps prevent illnesses and parasites and encourages good overall health. Whether your animals are on pasture or in a suburban backyard, it's possible to give them healthy herbs and treats that will encourage a natural diet and lifestyle. And it's also very possible to make your own tinctures and supplements for your livestock that are in many cases more effective than the chemical ones.

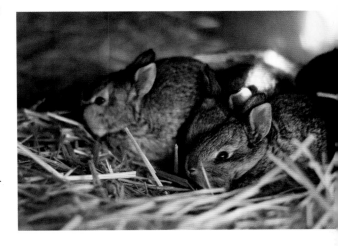

Whether giving your livestock herbal supplements, herbs in their feed (wild-foraged or added), or having an herbal medicine cabinet ready to go, you'll find that your livestock is the healthiest it has ever been.

ADDING HERBS TO LIVESTOCK FEED

If you have large livestock or just a few smaller animals like rabbits, herbs can be added to your favorite livestock feed to help enhance the health of your animals. Yes, it's even possible to do this in the feed of chickens that never touch pasture. Even large poultry companies are adding oregano and thyme to their chicken feeds as natural antibiotics. (We'll go into more detail on chickens and their herbal needs in the next chapter.)

As a general rule, when I mix up my bags of feed with herbs, I try not to make the herbs more than 10 to 15 percent of the feed. But my animals also forage naturally. You may find that in the winter months, you add different herbs (or more herbs) than you would in the summer . . . and so on. You can rotate different herb mixes with each and every new batch you make. Refer to the homesteader's herb list at the beginning of the book (chapter 2) to see which herbs you'd like to add to your livestock feed, keeping in mind that some herbs aren't good for certain livestock, though most herbs can be given in small amounts.

Here is a list of herbs that I add to my livestock feed that are generally good for all livestock. Many of these herbs can be found in the wild or in your garden, or you can purchase them online. You can offer them fresh or dried. As always, I do encourage you to choose herbs wisely when offering them to pregnant livestock.

Herbs for livestock feed

Chicory	Thyme	Nasturtium	St. John's Wort
Plantain Leaf	Oregano	Sage	Lemon Balm
Garlic	Peppermint	Nettle	Calendula
Onion			

If nothing else, I am a strong advocate for adding garlic, oregano, and thyme to your livestock feed. These herbs can be eaten by all of your barnyard livestock, including pregnant livestock, and should be your main foundation for herbal feed. All of these help prevent viral and bacterial issues, stimulate the immune system, help rid the body of parasites, and encourage general overall health.

HERBS FOR LIVESTOCK PASTURE

One of the most overlooked opportunities for getting herbs into your livestock's daily diet is to add herbs to your pasture. Several years back, I visited a local farm that planted radishes, turnips, and other root vegetables throughout their pasture seed mix where their pigs wild-foraged. I had an "ah-ha" moment and thought to myself, *Why can't we do this with herbs?*

To my surprise, this method is popular throughout Australia and Europe. In the 1950s, English farmer Newman Turner wrote a book specifically about using herbs and natural wild foraging plants to aid in livestock fertility and health on his rotating pastures. The herbs, combined with pasture rotation, made for extremely healthy and happy livestock.

Today, we can implement these same methods. In fact, we see internationally known farmers, like Joel Salatin, teaching about these pasture-raising methods on a regular basis.

Not only are herbs in your pasture grass beneficial to the animals, they're also beneficial to maintain and build healthy soil. Herbs help prevent soil erosion because they have deep root systems. Once established, your pasture will bless you and your livestock year after year because the perennial herbs grow deeper and deeper with each new season. Herbs are also great in pastures where you cut hay, as they offer dried herbs throughout the entire winter to your livestock.

Keep in mind that you want to keep a balance in all things. If your pasture has a predominance of herbs like chicory, this could come through in the taste and smell of your dairy.

Beneficial pasture herbs

Chicory	Oregano	St. John's Wort	Peppermint
Parsley	Lambs Quarter	Red Raspberry	Chamomile
Chickweed	Mullein	Burdock	Yarrow
Plantain	Dandelion	Nettle	Red Clover
Thyme	Calendula	Lemon Balm	Birdsfoot Trefoil

When planting seeds, allow your pasture to get established before turning out your livestock. Grazing your livestock for a week and then rotating between new pastures or paddocks for 1–4 weeks really helps keep all pastures healthy and in continuous growth with healthy root systems intact.

LIVESTOCK HERBAL PRODUCTS

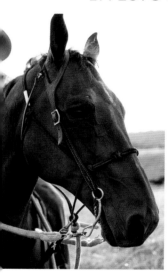

Offering our livestock free choice of herbs in their feed and on pasture is so essential to their good health. But even if we do this and keep the barn as clean as a whistle, things still happen. They might sustain a flesh wound from another goat's horn, get caught in barbed wire, or have worms or intestinal parasites. The list is endless. In fact, in the world of farming and homesteading, we often say, "If something *can* go wrong, it *will* go wrong."

As with your own family, tinctures, salves, ointments, and other herbal products can come to the rescue. Some of them you'll need to make in advance and keep on hand, while others you can make up quickly with products you may already have. Let's walk through each of the following recipes and talk about how it works.

Herbal Healing Salve

An herbal healing salve can be used on even the smallest of livestock, like rabbits and chickens. Use this healing salve on wounds, skin irritations, and other external areas that need cleansing and quick soothing. The oregano and manuka honey in this salve give it antiseptic and antibacterial properties, allowing the wound to

stay free of infection. Apply this salve directly on the affected area.
(See infused oil recipes on page 146.)

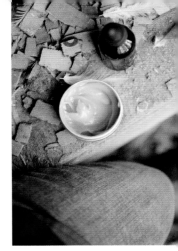

1 oz chamomile-infused oil

1 oz oregano-infused oil

1 oz calendula-infused oil

.5 oz beeswax

1 tbsp manuka honey

METHOD:

1. Create a double boiler by filling a saucepan with about 1–2 inches of water and putting a mason jar in the saucepan. Bring the water to a simmer.

2. In the mason jar, add the infused oils and beeswax. Melt completely.

3. Remove from heat and add the manuka honey. Combine well.

4. Pour into salve tins or keep in the mason jar until ready to use. Cap it tightly after it has cooled completely, label it, and store for 6–12 months or until it has lost most of its aroma.

Black Drawing Salve (see page 150 for recipe)

We use black drawing salve for a lot of things, but I especially enjoy using it on rooster combs. In the wintertime, sometimes chicken combs will get specks (or more) of frostbite, depending on the breed. I once asked an older farmer what he used to heal the frostbite and deter the chickens from pecking at each other. He suggested purchasing the over-the-counter livestock-grade Ichthammol from the farm store. I used it, and it worked well, but in the back of my mind, I knew I could make an herbal alternative. And so, this homemade black drawing salve was created. You can use essential oils or infused oils in the recipe. It can be used on both livestock and your human family. Use it on chicken combs, wounds, bumblefoot, and more.

Wound Spray

We all know the big name brands make claims that their wound sprays are all natural and can be used on open wounds, for pink eye, and other animal ailments. But what you may not realize is that many of these sprays don't have a single herb in them. While their ingredients may be natural, they are still very much man-made.

We can make our own herbal alternatives on our homestead for our animals with great success, including this spray, which helps heal open wounds, irritations, fungal infections, and more. Smaller batches can be made if you won't be using this amount of product within two days. **Note:** Please don't use this recipe for pink eye, as the aloe vera and other herbs could cause a reaction with the eye.

water

2 oz goldenseal (or Oregon grape root), dried

3 oz comfrey, dried

3 oz chamomile, dried

1 tbsp aloe vera gel (optional)

2 tbsp raw honey

10 drops tea tree essential oil

5 drops frankincense essential oil (optional)

10 drops myrrh essential oil (optional)

METHOD:

1. In a saucepan, boil 4 cups of water and then allow to cool slightly.

2. In a 16-ounce spray bottle, add goldenseal, comfrey, and chamomile. Pour in aloe vera gel and honey.

3. Pour the warm water into the bottle over the herbs, filling all the way to the top leaving some headspace. Add essential oils once water has cooled. Shake well.

4. Spray on wounds and other external areas of your animal that need healing. Keep away from eyes. Use within two days.

Herbal Pink Eye Solution

While the wound spray is amazing and effective, it's not best for the eyes and can cause irritation. Use this simple herbal remedy to heal pink eye and make your own pink eye solution and compresses. This can be used for animals and humans! This mixture should be used within 24 hours. Making a new batch is super easy, and it's why we like to use small spray bottles for this treatment.

1–2 tbsp raw honey (or manuka honey)
.5 oz chamomile tea
1 smashed garlic clove
distilled water

METHOD:

1. Add 1–2 tablespoons of raw honey into a 1-ounce spray bottle.

2. Fill the bottle about halfway up with chamomile tea. Add garlic clove.

3. Fill the remaining portion of the bottle with distilled water.

4. Shake well, then spray onto affected livestock eyes, concentrating around the eye itself. Or use compresses to clean the eye each day. Keeping the eye clean with this solution is key.

Horses and black walnut hulls

It is extremely important to note that horses have a much more complex health system than most four-legged livestock. For this reason, I *highly* suggest consulting with a veterinarian before administering any type of herbal remedy to horses. This includes the black walnut hulls used in the following recipe. Horses typically only have an issue with black walnut tree shavings, but further studies are needed when it comes to the hulls. For this reason, the dosage for horses should be less than the dosage for other livestock.

Herbal Livestock Parasite Tincture

My husband had the brilliant idea of getting meat rabbits when we first started our homesteading journey. And then I had the brilliant idea of expanding our rabbitry until I could barely tend to it myself. The first time a litter of our rabbits got an internal parasite, it just about sent me overboard.

I used an over-the-counter tincture that I found online. We still lost the entire litter.

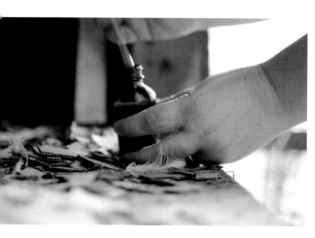

It was then that I realized just how important parasitic prevention is. Prevention is key with herbs, and with rotating your livestock on pasture. Since then, I've created my own tincture that has proven to work time and time again. We use this tincture as a preventative once a week, or once every other week. Our rabbits haven't gotten parasites since. When it's not typically wet outside, I drop it down to once a month.

If parasites were to ever arise, which they haven't, I would give the tincture four times each day for 2–4 weeks.

Be advised that the amount of vodka used in this tincture, and all tinctures, is so minute that it won't affect your animals in any way whatsoever. Please use caution when administering to horses (see sidebar on page 263).

.5 oz clove, ground

.5 oz black walnut hulls, ground (or powdered)

1 oz thyme

1 oz grapefruit seed

2 garlic cloves

15 oz 80 proof vodka

METHOD:

1. Premeasure all herbs and vodka.

2. In a large glass jar, add all herbs. Cover the herbs with the entire 15 ounces of vodka. They may not be completely submerged, but that's okay.

3. Shake your tincture liberally and then set it in a cool pantry or cupboard, away from extreme temperature changes and direct sunlight. Shake your tincture each day (multiple times, if you want) for four weeks.

4. After 4–6 weeks, strain your tincture from the jar. Pour your strained tincture into a colored glass eyedropper bottle, label, and store in a cool place until ready to use.

5. Use tincture as a preventative once a month by mouth or in livestock waterer, according to your own schedule. If parasites arise, use once every 4 hours for 2–4 weeks.

Tincture dosage for livestock

1 eyedropper (30 drops) per 150 lbs • 50–75 lbs (15 drops) • 25–45 lbs (5 to 10 drops)

Make dosage according to weight ratio of 150 lbs for 25 lbs or less

When in doubt, start with 5 drops and work up from there. It's okay to start small!

Herbal Livestock Worming Tincture

This tincture can be given for 1–2 weeks at the first sign of worms. Adjust the liquid ratio accordingly. At the first sign of worms or parasites, give the tincture twice a day for two weeks.

1 oz ginger root
1 oz plantain leaf
2 cloves garlic
.25 oz black walnut hulls
16 oz 80 proof vodka

METHOD:

1. Premeasure all herbs and vodka.

2. In a large glass jar, add all herbs. Cover the herbs with the entire 16 oz of vodka. They may not be completely submerged, but that's okay.

3. Shake your tincture liberally and then set it in a cool pantry or cupboard, away from extreme temperature changes and direct sunlight. Shake your tincture each day (multiple times, if you want) for four weeks.

4. After 4–6 weeks, strain your tincture from the jar. Pour your strained tincture into a colored glass eyedropper bottle, label, and store in a cool place until ready to use. Administer directly by mouth if treating just a few animals or by waterer if treating an entire herd.

Antibacterial and Antiviral Tincture

If you have no other tincture for your livestock on hand, make sure you have this one. It works great as a preventative when you've brought a new animal to the farm. It is also an aggressive tincture against bacterial and viral issues.

1 oz echinacea (root or leaves)

.5 oz Oregon grape root

.5 oz thyme

.5 oz oregano

2 smashed garlic cloves

10 oz 80 proof vodka or glycerin

METHOD:

1. Add all herbs to a glass jar and cover with 10 ounces of vodka or glycerin.

2. Cap tightly and set in a dark, temperature-controlled space (like a pantry or cupboard) for 4–6 weeks. Shake tincture 1–2 times each day (morning and evening work well).

3. After 4–6 weeks, strain tincture into a glass eyedropper bottle. Label and store in medicine cabinet or cupboard. Administer directly by mouth if treating just a few animals or by waterer if treating an entire herd.

Notes: If using as a preventative, make a separate tincture without the Oregon grape root, as it should not be used as a preventative.

Herbal Lice and External Parasite Spray

Lice, mites, and other external parasites are from the devil, of this I am sure. They are the worst things to get rid of. This oil mixture has been proven to help sheep, goats, and cattle. You can spray the oil directly on the skin of the animal, or add drops down the back line. You'll need to do it 1–2 times a day for two weeks. In between sprays, you can also use diatomaceous earth and neem powder on your livestock's skin to kill parasites directly. **Note:** Do not use on chickens or cats, as it can be toxic to cats, and it's not very effective on chickens.

2 oz neem oil or olive oil

7 drops tea tree essential oil

7 drops rosemary essential oil

7 drops eucalyptus essential oil

witch hazel (1 part)

distilled water (3 parts)

1-oz spray bottle

METHOD:

1. Mix all ingredients in a spray bottle. Shake well.

2. Shake before each use. Spray directly on the skin of the animal, concentrating on the back line and around the neck. Repeat once in the morning and once in the evening, if necessary. Continue use for two weeks until lice and parasites are gone.

Soothing Udder Balm

Sometimes a homesteader's goats and milk cows need extra love and care on their udders. This salve is a fabulous recipe to help soothe and heal the udder, and is safe for younger livestock that may still be nursing on mama.

1 oz calendula-infused oil

1 oz plantain-infused oil

1 oz chamomile-infused oil

1 oz shea butter

1 tsp lanolin (optional)

.5 oz beeswax

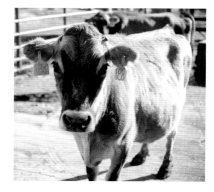

METHOD:

1. Create a double boiler with a saucepan filled with 1–2 inches of water and a mason jar.

2. In the mason jar, add the infused oils, shea butter, lanolin, and beeswax. Melt completely.

3. Pour into salve into tins or keep in the mason jar until ready to use. Cap it tightly after it has cooled completely, label, and store for 6–12 months or until it has lost most of its aroma. Use as needed.

Herbal Udder Wash

We can spend an unreasonable amount of money on purchasing udder washes. Why do that when making your own udder wash is incredibly easy, quick, and affordable? Here's a simple recipe that you can make up in a jiffy. Just make sure you're using therapeutic grade essential oils, not the fragrance oils you buy from a big-box store.

10 drops clove essential oil

15 drops tea tree essential oil

15 drops lavender essential oil

1 tbsp alcohol

1–2 tbsp castile soap (optional)

distilled water

METHOD:

1. In a 16-ounce glass spray bottle, add essential oils and alcohol.

2. If you are adding castile soap, add it at this point.

3. Fill the rest of the bottle up with distilled water. Shake well.

4. Shake bottle well before each use. Spray as needed and wipe clean before milking.

Essential oils for livestock

There has been some debate as to whether or not essential oils (EOs) can be used on livestock. I'm here to tell you that they absolutely can be. While we don't suggest the ingestion of essential oils with livestock, animals do react well to topical and aromatic applications of EOs. Here are some examples:

Respiratory Blend: peppermint, eucalyptus, tea tree, lemon, and cardamom

Digestive Blend: ginger, peppermint, tarragon, fennel, and anise

Pest Control Blend: tea tree, peppermint, and eucalyptus

Chickens: 1–2 drops under wings

Large Livestock: 2–3 drops on skin of neck

HERBS FOR THE HOMESTEAD DOG

My biggest "ah-ha" moment in terms of farm dogs came from watching our Black Mouth Cur named Delilah. She had come down with a urinary tract infection, as many female dogs do. I had given her one antibiotic capsule but, hours later, I noticed she was outside chowing down on my echinacea plants.

I began to freak out a bit. My precious echinacea was being destroyed by a crazy dog. After noticing that each time she went outside she'd start eating echinacea leaves, I realized that nature was actually at work right in front of me. Delilah was self-medicating.

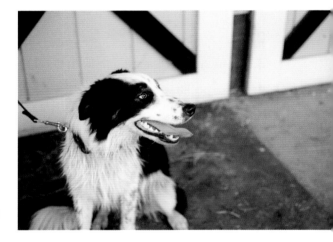

Because Delilah is closer to a wild dog in the gene pool than our goofy Labrador Retriever, Samson, she hasn't completely lost touch with nature like he has after years of breeding for conformation.

I didn't give Delilah any more antibiotics and watched her closely. She rested frequently, ate echinacea three times a day on her own, and within seven days she was completely healed. As an herbalist, I felt honored to have witnessed this so closely firsthand.

This simply proved my theory that if given the proper natural tools, animals can heal themselves in many situations. While I lost three echinacea plants in the process, I witnessed something far greater at work.

The Native Americans used echinacea as a natural antibiotic, something we often don't think of when it comes to how we use it today. But very clearly, it can be just as effective today as it was back then. At least, Delilah thought so, and she was right.

Herbs in Dog Food and Treats

We don't give our dogs herbs every single day. A few times a week seems to be the norm. I find myself adding garlic powder, turmeric powder, and powdered echinacea leaves to their bowls most often. We found that switching them over to a completely grain-free diet helped eliminate a lot of their former health issues. There are many herbs you can offer your canine friends throughout the week—you can sprinkle these herbs, fresh or dried, in their feed, or make snacks out of them. Keep in mind that a little bit of these herbs goes a long way and sometimes powdered is best.

Herbs for dogs

Peppermint	Sage	Astragalus
Oregano	Ginger	St. John's
Rosemary	Turmeric	Wort
Basil	Dandelion	Chamomile
Thyme	Echinacea	Lavender
Garlic		

Herbal Dog Treats

You can purchase herbal dog treats online, but why not make them at home? Your pups will love these treats and get an immunity boost all at the same time.

1 cup pumpkin puree

3 tbsp coconut oil

1 farm fresh egg

1½ cups einkorn flour (or a gluten-free flour)

½ oz astragalus root, powdered

½ oz echinacea root, powdered

2 tsp garlic powder

METHOD:

1. Preheat oven to 300°F.

2. Combine pumpkin puree, coconut oil, and egg in a bowl. Set aside.

3. Combine flour and herbs in a separate bowl, then combine with wet mixture. Mix completely. Mixture should feel moist but not too wet.

4. Roll out to about ¼-inch thickness and cut into treat shapes.

5. Bake on a lined baking sheet for 20–30 minutes, or until crispy. Let cool completely.

6. Store in an airtight container in the pantry or fridge for up to two weeks. They will last longer in the fridge.

Dehydrated Meat Dog Treats

Dehydrating thin slices of meat, liver, heart, or other organs from chickens, venison, bison, or beef can prove to be a very effective way of administering herbs to your farm dog. Play around with some of the herbs and meats mentioned in this recipe.

2 oz of powdered herbs (see sidebar on page 273)

1–2 lbs meat or animal organ of choice

METHOD:

1. Preheat dehydrator to 155°F.

2. Mix up herbs in a container.

3. Cut meat into ¼-inch slices. Douse each piece in the powdered herbs.

4. Lay in a single layer on dehydrator racks. Dry for 6–8 hours or until crispy. They may be slightly leathery, but must be completely dry all the way through.

5. Store in an airtight container for up to six months. Store in freezer for up to one year.

Meats to use for dog treats	Powdered herbs to use for dog treats
Chicken	Garlic
Venison	Turmeric
Bison	Oregano
Turkey	Thyme
Fish	Basil
Beef	Parsley
Squirrel	Ginger
Rabbit	Sage
Internal Livestock Organs (liver, heart, tongue)	Rosemary
	Echinacea

Farm Dog Herbal Treatment Products

Our dogs are constantly running about without a care in the world, which normally means they don't realize they've cut their foot or have fleas all over them until it's too late. We breathed a sigh of relief when we realized there were homemade products that worked just as well as over-the-counter ones. Here are some products you may want to keep on hand, or at least in mind, for your farmstead dog.

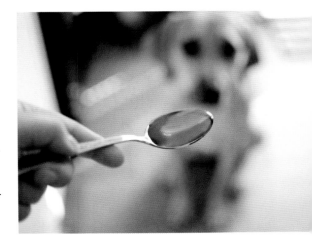

Ear Mite Treatment

This treatment can be used on any animal. It is simple and easy, and something we especially used on our rabbits when they needed help with ear mites. This also works well for ear yeast infections. If choosing to use the garlic in this recipe, you'll need to make this honey treatment ahead of time. You can choose not to use the garlic and just create a honey and water mixture. It works fine as well.

3 cloves garlic, smashed

2 oz raw honey (or manuka honey)

distilled water

METHOD:

1. Infuse garlic in honey for two weeks in a sunny window. Once infused, strain out garlic and transfer the honey to a pantry. Label container.

2. When ready to use, mix the infused honey with a little water so that it makes the honey thinner. Put a few drops at a time on the inside of the animal's ear, enough so that the honey covers the inside of the ear from top to bottom, but not in excess. Massage the ear to ensure that it gets down into the ear canal. Continue to treat for 7–14 days.

Flea and Insect Repellent Spray

Here's an herbal alternative to chemical flea and insect repellent sprays. We use this whenever we go for a walk or let the dogs out to play.

distilled water

10 drops eucalyptus essential oil

7 drops lavender essential oil

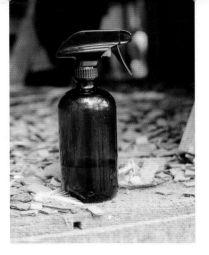

10 drops tea tree essential oil

5 drops oregano essential oil

5 drops citronella essential oil (optional)

witch hazel

METHOD:

1. Fill a 16-ounce glass spray bottle three-quarters of the way with distilled water.

2. Add essential oils.

3. Fill remaining part of the bottle with witch hazel (about ¼ cup).

4. Shake well and spray lightly on the feet of your pets and on their back lines. Be sure not to get it in their ears or eyes. Apply as needed.

Flea-Be-Gone Bath Soap
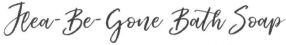

Many people don't realize that any lathering soap will kill fleas. Whether it's a dish liquid or a castile soap, they will both get the job done. We opt for a castile soap and add a few essential oils to it to get the job completely done. This shouldn't be used every week, as you can dry out your dog's skin if it's used too often, but it can be used once every 6–8 weeks or more.

3 cups castile soap

3 drops lavender essential oil

3 drops oregano essential oil

2 drops tea tree essential oil

2 drops eucalyptus essential oil

METHOD:

1. In a glass bottle, mix all ingredients together, stirring well to incorporate oils.

2. Use as necessary, making sure you lather the soap on your dog right down to the skin. It needs to come in contact with the skin to be most effective. A little bit goes a long way.

3. Wash pet thoroughly. Use mixture up within six months.

Tea Tree Healing Honey

One day our Lab Samson left a trail of bloody footprints across the floor I had just mopped—isn't that always the way? I quickly realized Samson needed something antibacterial, and it needed to be something I had on hand. I cleaned the wounded area well and then added this mixture to the cut. I sat with him for about 5–10 minutes, ensuring that he didn't lick the area while the healing honey was doing its work. Wrapping the affected area or wiping it clean after the 10-minute time period is best. Afterwards, I let him at it. I would simply have to reapply the honey every few hours. He healed within four days, and we were back to normal!

1 tbsp raw honey (or manuka honey, or chamomile- or thyme-infused honey)

5 drops tea tree essential oil

2 drops oregano essential oil

METHOD:

1. In a small jar, mix together honey and essential oils.

2. Place mixture liberally on affected area and allow to set without being disturbed for 10 minutes.

3. Apply every 4 hours or as needed, until wound closes up completely.

Is tea tree oil toxic to dogs?

It's debated whether tea tree essential oil is toxic when it comes to dogs. Let's face it, anything can be toxic to the body in high dosages. Tea tree essential oil contains phenolic compounds that can be hard for a dog's body to process. But for a dog to reach toxic levels of tea tree oil (whether ingested or given externally), it would have to receive .22 grams of oil per 1 pound of body weight. That means a 1-pound dog would have to receive 4 drops of tea tree essential oil before it would begin to have toxic effects. If you have a 10-pound dog, you'd have to use more than 40 drops of tea tree oil to reach toxic levels, and so on. To err on the side of caution, only use tea tree essential oil externally. It's important to note that tea tree essential oil should not be used on cats or animals smaller than 10 pounds. And tea tree oil should never be used for an extended period of time.

Urinary Tract Infection Tincture

Female dogs can have one heck of a time with urinary tract infections. Instead of slipping off to the doctor for an antibiotic every single time, try this herbal tincture for your beloved farm dog!

.5 oz cranberry powder

1 oz echinacea root (or crushed leaves, dried)

2 cloves smashed garlic

7 oz 80 proof vodka

METHOD:

1. In a glass jar, add powder and herbs and cover completely with vodka.

2. Cap jar, shake well, and set in a temperature-controlled pantry or cabinet, out of direct sunlight, for 4–6 weeks. Shake the mixture each day, once in the morning and once in the evening.

3. After 4–6 weeks of extraction, strain tincture into a glass eyedropper bottle. Cap tightly and label. Store in medicine cabinet or pantry.

4. Administer three times a day until symptoms disappear.

Tincture dosages for dogs

1 eyedropper (30 drops) per 150 lbs • 50–75 lbs (10 drops) • 25–45 lbs (7 drops)

Make dosage according to weight ratio for 25 lbs or less

Deworming Tincture

Worms come in all different shapes, kinds, and sizes. Use this tincture to rid your dog of worms and internal parasites. Each herb used has a specific worm that it helps expel. The milk thistle seed helps protect the liver and other organs from the black walnut hull tannins.

.5 oz black walnut hulls

.75 oz milk thistle seed

.25 oz chamomile

1 garlic clove, smashed

7.5 oz 80 proof vodka

METHOD:

1. Place all herbs in a glass jar.

2. Cover herbs with 7.5 ounces of vodka. Cap and shake well.

3. Set in a temperature-controlled area, like a pantry or cabinet, out of direct sunlight for 4–6 weeks.

4. After 4–6 weeks, strain out herbs and pour tincture into a glass eyedropper bottle. Label and store in medicine cabinet.

5. Administer orally three times a day for two weeks.

Herbs are so versatile that they can be used for just about any animal. Now that I've gone over most of the four-legged creatures you may have roaming your property, we can move on to other animals, like chickens and bees, both of which benefit from herbs more than we may realize.

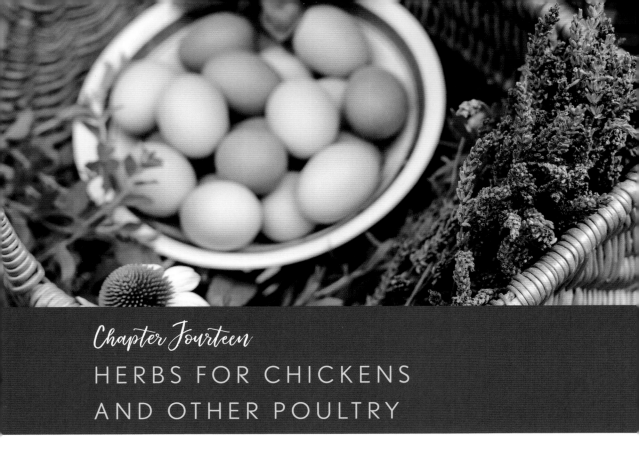

Chapter Fourteen

HERBS FOR CHICKENS AND OTHER POULTRY

Chickens are taking over the world! Homesteaders love their chickens, and so does every suburban family out there. Many people in subdivisions can't have large livestock, so they opt for chickens or other poultry. They are extremely easy to maintain if you only have a few. And ultimately, it isn't very difficult to keep them healthy if they are given the proper habitat and preventatives.

I could probably write an entire book about chickens myself, but as a homesteader, I just need the basics, and I'm sure you're that way as well. For most of us, we love the heck out of our chickens, but we don't need to go too far into the pampering part. Please, don't ever dress your chickens up. Get what I mean? I know you do. While chickens are the most common of livestock on a homestead, they can often be the most complex and needy when it comes to their health. Offering your chickens, first and foremost, rotational grazing and free choice herbs is the best way to maintain a healthy lifestyle for the chicken. But sometimes things just happen. Let's walk through the herbal world of chickens.

We can be confident in our poultry endeavors when we offer herbs and other supplements by adding it to their feed or by giving free choice herbs. We can put herbs in their nesting boxes, herb bundles in the coop, and so on.

IN THE FEED, IN THE WATERER, OR FREE CHOICE HERBS

There are two main ways that I like to give herbs to my poultry: in their feed or in their waterers. I give them preventative herbs in their feed a couple times each week, but when I need to treat them, I go straight to the waterer with an infusion or tea. This ensures that my entire flock is treated.

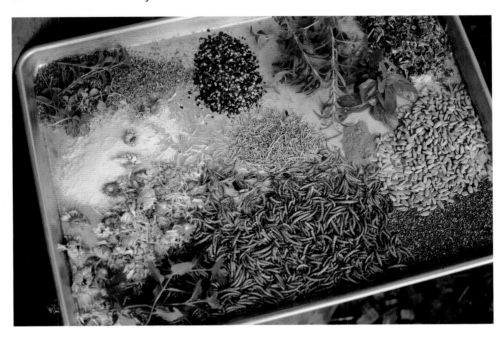

Preventative poultry feed and free choice herbs

Thyme: Has antibacterial and antibiotic properties, and also aids in respiratory health. It is even used by commercial chicken houses in the United States in place of harsh antibiotics.

Astragalus: Is a hard-core immune-boosting herb.

Oregano: Has antibacterial and antibiotic properties, and has an extremely high antioxidant content. It fights off infections and helps rid the body of infections.

Garlic: Naturally boosts the immune system and is a powerful bacteria fighter.

Turmeric: Is a natural anti-inflammatory with antioxidant properties that benefit the feathers and skin of poultry.

Sage: Aids in proper digestion and is great for the reproductive system.

Basil: Has anti-inflammatory and antioxidant properties, aids in proper digestion, and is just a fun treat!

Calendula: Is high in vitamins, and the color of calendula enhances the yolk of the chicken egg.

Herbal Teas and Infusions for the Waterer

There are several different ways you can infuse your poultry waterer with herbs, but no matter which way you choose to do it, make sure you clean out the waterer every 12–18 hours. Infusions like this lose their potency after that time period, and at that point your chickens are basically just drinking flavored water. Here are two ways to infuse your poultry waterer:

Infusion. As we learned in chapter 6, an infusion is when you use cold or boiling water to steep herbs. You can make infusions for your waterers by simply placing the herbs in the waterer and filling it with water. Or you can steep the herbs for 5 minutes in hot water to make a concentrate, and then add it to your waterer.

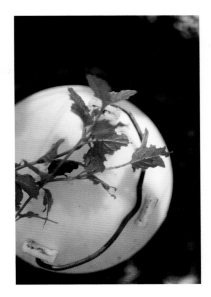

Decoction. Again, as we learned earlier, decoctions are a lot like infusions, except in order to extract the herbal benefits of the herb, the herb must be boiled, not just steeped in boiling water. This method is used for root herbs, seeds, barks, and herbs that are hard or come in thick casings. Make a decoction by boiling the herbs in a nonaluminum saucepan for 20 minutes, then add to a waterer of cold water. All of the following infusions are based on a one-gallon waterer or jug. You can make a gallon and put into smaller waterers for poultry like quail. Or you can just cut the batch by half.

Immunity-Boost Infusion

4 garlic cloves, smashed

.5 oz thyme, dried or wilted

.5 oz oregano, dried or wilted

METHOD:

Add all herbs to waterer, cover with fresh new water. Discard after 12–18 hours and make a new batch if needed.

Antibacterial and Antiviral Decoction

Poultry enthusiasts probably fear the avian flu more than anything. And really, an outbreak is something to be terrified of. But we can help pull our chickens through by preventing the flu from even coming into our flock by offering this decoction once a month for 5–7 days during migrations of birds that carry the avian flu. This decoction is also great when it comes to bacterial, viral, and parasitic issues in our poultry. In fact, astragalus root, the main herb in this decoction, has been clinically proven in a controlled study to not only prevent avian flu but to heal or shorten avian flu much more rapidly than chemical alternatives. It has also been shown to prevent the flu from being spread to other flock members when given as a preventative. This is also a fabulous decoction for mycoplasma and other chronic illnesses in chickens. At the Fewell homestead, we make a tincture out of these ingredients for a more aggressive treatment if necessary, though we've never had to use it, thankfully.

.25 oz elderberry

.25 oz ginger root

1 oz astragalus root

1 garlic clove

2–3 cups water

.25 oz thyme

METHOD:

1. Boil elderberries, ginger root, astragalus root, and garlic clove for 20 minutes in 2–3 cups of water to make a decoction.

2. Pour mixture over the thyme.

3. Pour 1–2 tablespoons of the decoction into waterer as necessary.

Summertime Cool-Down Infusion

Chickens can become stressed out in the summer months. This cooling infusion will help them through the heat!

½ cup fresh mint (peppermint or spearmint)

½ cup fresh basil

the peel from 1 lemon

METHOD:

Add all herbs into a fresh waterer. Replace every 12–18 hours or as needed.

Winter Warming Infusion

I don't do this infusion often, but when we have big winter storms, it's hard not to offer my flock something soothing. I usually warm the water before taking it out to them, as sometimes it's so cold that the water freezes as soon as I put it down. The cayenne in this infusion cannot be tasted by the chickens, but still gives them an internal warming effect and also helps rid their bodies of any wintertime issues that may be lurking. The chamomile soothes, and the cloves bring that added sense of cleanliness to the coop and the chickens with the scent of the herb.

.25 oz chamomile

3 whole cloves or 1 tsp clove powder

1 tsp ginger powder

1 tsp cayenne

boiling water

METHOD:

1. Place herbs in a jar and pour boiling water over top, just enough to cover them. Allow to set for 5–10 minutes, then add to a slightly warmed chicken waterer.

2. Replace every 12–18 hours.

Immunity, Antibacterial, and Antiviral Tincture

I often try to treat or prevent illness in my flocks through their feed and water infusions or decoctions first. But sometimes, it just doesn't work, and I have to resort to using tinctures. My favorite tincture to keep on hand works multiple ways. I haven't had to use it in more than five years since implementing preventative herbs, but it's still something I like to keep on hand if I bring home a chicken or duck from an auction or an unknown source. I'll give it as a preventative for a couple of days before the bird leaves quarantine. You can also use this tincture as an aggressive action toward respiratory and other bacterial and viral conditions. **Note:** Avoid giving to cows and horses, as there have not been enough studies done on the effects of astragalus with these animals. If absolutely necessary, use under the direction of your veterinarian.

Dosage for poultry: 2–5 drops (2 drops for 3 lbs and below, 5 drops for 4–8 lbs)

.5 oz dried astragalus root

.5 oz dried ginger root (or powder)

.5 oz thyme

.5 oz oregano

2 g clove

10 oz 80 proof vodka or glycerin

METHOD:

1. Add all herbs to a glass jar and cover with 10 ounces of vodka or glycerin.

2. Cap tightly and set in a dark, temperature-controlled space (like a pantry or cupboard) for 4–6 weeks. Shake tincture 1–2 times each day (morning and evening work well).

3. After 4–6 weeks, strain tincture into a glass eyedropper bottle. Label and store in medicine cabinet or cupboard. Tincture will keep for several years, but check it frequently after the first year.

IN THE NESTING BOX

While it's not something I do all of the time, adding fresh or dried herbs to nesting boxes can help freshen up the coop in the summer months. Adding an herbal nesting box mix to your nesting boxes brings a sense of calm to the chaos, especially for broodies, but is mostly just a natural way to spruce up your chicken coop. Fresh herbs, however, are great for chick brooders, as the natural oils help inhibit bacteria growth. You can make up a batch of dried herbs throughout the year, or

Nesting box herbs

Chamomile	Comfrey
Calendula	Dill
Yarrow	Mint
Basil	Nasturtium
Oregano	Rosemary
Thyme	Plantain Leaf
Lemon Balm	Sage

use fresh herbs in the summer months when you have them readily available. As always, keep a clean coop and nesting box for ultimate and efficient laying. There's no rhyme or reason to mixing these herbs. Just throw in whatever you have in abundance and let it go to work!

IN THE DUST BATH

As we well know, avoiding things like external parasites begins with healthy animals and prevention. Given the proper natural tools, livestock can tend to themselves. One of these tools is the dust bath that your chickens bathe in on a weekly basis. We can add herbs and other natural ingredients to their dust bath to help rid them of parasites and lice. Here are the herbs and natural products we use in our dust bathing area:

Turmeric powder	Rosemary	Diatomaceous Earth
Garlic powder	Chamomile	Wood Ash
Mint		

Herbs in the chick brooder

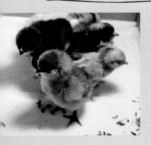

Even the newest flock members can benefit from herbs in their feed and brooder! Offer free choice herbs like thyme, oregano, and garlic to your chicks to help boost their immune systems and prevent coccidiosis. Infuse the herbs into their waterer for an added boost of immune-stimulating properties. Or sprinkle fresh herbs around the brooder to help keep down parasites and other unwanted nasties.

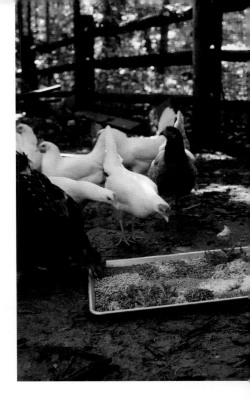

Chickens are the drama queens of the homestead, but they greatly benefit from preventative herbs. One of my most closely held beliefs is that, if given the proper tools, our smaller livestock can live healthy lives as naturally as possible. With little effort, we can offer our chickens and other poultry opportunities that encourage free ranging, enhance and promote orange egg yolks, and in return, benefit us as homesteaders.

Along with all of these amazing herbs you might be growing for your chickens and your family, you'll also hear the buzz of bees. Let's take a look at our fearless pollinators in the next chapter, and learn how they make herbs possible for us, and ultimately, how our herb gardens benefit bees in the long run.

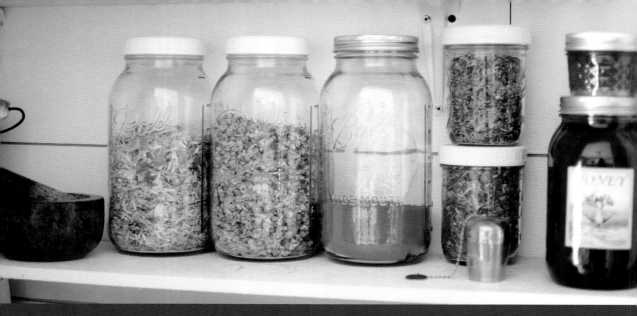

Chapter Fifteen

MY HERBAL MEDICINE CABINET AND PANTRY

We can talk about how to use herbs, where to use them, and what to make with them all day long but, when it comes right down to it, most people just want a handy reference of what to keep in the pantry and medicine cabinet.

I get it. I want to know the basics too. *Just tell me how to do it already!*

Sometimes, it's easier to mimic the methods of another person when we first start out. As we grow, we adapt the methods and make them our own. It's easy to get caught up in the thousands of herbs that are out there, when in reality, we may only need twenty of them in our homes.

Beside herbs, what products does a homesteading herbalist need? These are things like eyedropper bottles, funnels, a kitchen scale, or extra muslin or cheesecloth for straining that we don't often think about keeping on hand.

I'll try to make all of this simple and painless for you. Let's go through all of the herbal things I like to have available for my family (hint: I don't keep everything in this book on hand at all times). I'll also go over the products you'll find in my home. Then, we'll go through my livestock herbal medicine cabinet, favorite gardening tools, and more!

WHAT'S IN MY HERBAL MEDICINE CABINET?

Here are the top things that I keep at all times (or most often) in my herbal medicine cabinet for my family.

Essential oils:

Cedarwood, Cinnamon, Clary Sage, Clove, Eucalyptus, Frankincense, Lavender, Lemon, Lemongrass, Myrrh, Oregano, Peppermint, Tea Tree, Vetiver, and various oil blends for respiratory ailments, hormonal balancing, and immune boosting.

Herbs (dried):

Arnica, Astragalus, Black Walnut Hull, Calendula, Cayenne, Chamomile, Curry, Echinacea, Elderberry, Garlic, Lavender, Lemon Balm, Mullein, Oregano, Peppermint, Rosemary, Thyme, Turmeric, Yarrow, Marshmallow, and various other herbs mentioned in this book, depending on the season.

Syrups and tinctures:

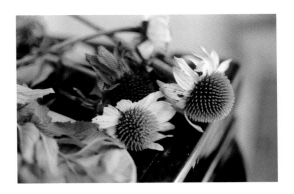

    Elderberry and Astragalus Syrup

    Elderberry, Astragalus, and Wild Cherry Bark Syrup

    Fire Cider

    Burdock Tincture

    Echinacea and Astragalus Tincture

    Milk Thistle Tincture

Teas:

Sleep-Encouraging Tea

Cough-Relief Tea

Salves and lotions:

Burn and Wound Healing Salve

Soothing Salve

Respiratory Salve

Antibacterial Ointment

Farmer's Hand Cream

Capsules:

Milk Thistle seed, powdered

Probiotics

Activated charcoal

Turmeric

Vitamins

Generic pain medicine (that's right, just in case!)

Empty capsules

Supplies:

Glass spray bottles (1-oz and 16-oz)

Glass eyedropper bottles (1-oz)

Various glass roll-on bottles for oil blends

Vodka (80 proof)

Glycerin

Witch Hazel

Raw (local or homegrown) honey

General first aid supplies

Essential oil diffuser

Half-gallon mason jars and screw-top lids

Pint mason jars and screw-top lids

Unbleached muslin for poultices and compresses

Thermometer

Pipettes

MY LIVESTOCK HERBAL MEDICINE CABINET

The herbal medicine cabinet for my livestock is pretty simple and straightforward. In herbalism, we find that multiple things can be eased or cured with the same herbs. With that said, here are the top things that I keep at all times (or most often) in my livestock herbal medicine cabinet.

Essential oils:

Frankincense, Peppermint, Oregano, Tea Tree, Thyme, Respiratory Blend

Herbs (dried):

Black Walnut Hulls, Cranberry, Comfrey, Elderberry, Garlic, Lavender, Nettle, Oregano, Red Raspberry Leaf, Thyme, Turmeric

Salves and sprays:

Black Drawing Salve

Herbal Healing Salve

Wound Spray

Soothing Udder Balm

Herbal Udder Wash

Tinctures:

Herbal Livestock Parasite Tincture

Herbal Livestock Worming Tincture

Immunity, Antibacterial, and Antiviral Tincture

Supplies:

Same as my homestead medicine cabinet, plus:

Self-adhesive bandage wraps	Syringes
Rubbing alcohol	Thermometer

MY FAVORITE GARDEN AND HERBALIST TOOLS AND PRODUCTS

I'm a woman who needs to keep things efficient in my life. I don't have time to go around trying every newfangled whatchamacallit product that gets sent my way. However, I have found some of my all-time favorite products this way, so I'm not going to complain. Some of them are about efficiency in the garden, while others are about nostalgia and comfort.

Here are some of my favorite tools to use in the garden, and some of the tools and products I keep on hand in the kitchen and for herb needs in general. You never know when you might want to cook up (or tincture up) with a batch of herbs!

In the garden:

My grandmother's wicker basket (handmade)

Sharp scissors

Hemp or jute twine

Carhartt work gloves and apparel

Lady Farmer apparel

Reformation Acres gathering apron

Sloggers work apron and boots

Generic overalls

Carhartt insulated overalls

Ducks Unlimited boots

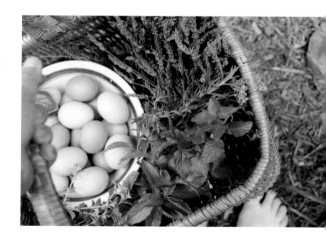

Hand pruner

Wheelbarrow

Trowel

Rototiller

Shovel

Push-pull hoe

Garden pick

Garden fence wire

T-posts

4-inch transplant pots

Soil blocker

Mason bee house

Neem oil (for garden bug pests)

Blood meal fertilizer

Materia medica journal (by *The Herbal Academy*)

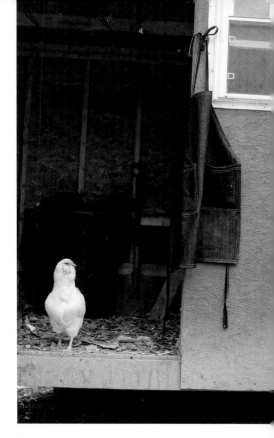

In the herbal kitchen and home:

Excalibur 5-drawer dehydrator

Half-waist bistro apron

Fluffy Layers apron

Indoor 5-shelf greenhouse

Various herb drying racks

Root storage bin (for ginger, turmeric, etc)

Mortar and pestle

Empty glass spice jars

Cast-iron skillets

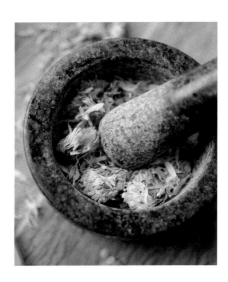

Dutch oven

Flip-top glass bottles and jars

Half-gallon mason jars and screw-top lids

Pint mason jars and screw-top lids

White vinegar

Apple cider vinegar (raw)

Cheesecloth

Cutting boards (wooden and glass)

Scissors

Hemp or jute twine

Afterword

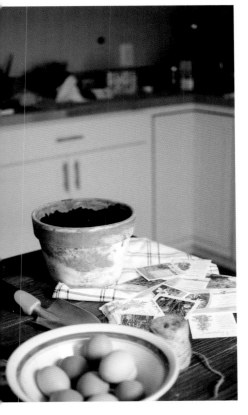

I started growing herbs because I wanted a simpler lifestyle, and so my journey of homesteading and becoming an herbal homesteader began.

We can spend hours and hours trying to learn everything there is to know about herbs and herbalism, but at the end of the day, it must be worth it. You don't have to know *all the things*, dear homesteader. Allow life to teach you naturally, and you'll retain so much more.

Whether you're a beginner or a seasoned herb gardener, take a deep breath and think of all the beauty that surrounds you. And at the end of the day, if it brings you peace, push forward with it. And if it doesn't, try again later.

Herbalism and gardening are hard work, but they are good work. And when you think you have no idea what you're doing, take notice, because then, and only then, can you truly begin to learn.

Resources and Further Learning

Here's a list of books, courses, and other things that I think you'll find of good use to further your herbal education. These are also resources that I've used myself while writing this book.

BOOKS:

Simple & Natural Soapmaking by Jan Berry

The Herb Book by John Lust

Rodale's Illustrated Encyclopedia of Herbs edited by Claire Kowalchik and William H. Hylton

The Handbook of Vintage Remedies by Jessie Hawkins

Modern Essentials, ninth edition, published by Aroma Tools

The Herbal Medicine-Maker's Handbook by James Green

Fertility Pastures by Newman Turner

Cure Your Own Cattle by Newman Turner

HERB SCHOOLS:

The Vintage Remedies Learning Center

http://www.vintageremedies.com

The Franklin Institute of Wellness

http://www.franklininstituteofwellness.com

The Herbal Academy

http://www.theherbalacademy.com

WHERE TO BUY ORGANIC HERBS, ESSENTIAL OILS, AND HERBAL PRODUCTS:

The Fewell Homestead

http://www.thefewellhomestead.com

dōTERRA

http://www.mydoterra.com/amyfewell

Bulk Herb Store

http://www.bulkherbstore.com

Mountain Rose Herbs

http://www.mountainroseherbs.com

Starwest Botanicals

http://www.starwest-botanicals.com

Baker Creek Heirloom Seeds

http://www.rareseeds.com

Seed Savers Exchange

http://www.seedsavers.org

WHERE TO BUY GARDENING/ HOMESTEADING SUPPLIES AND APPAREL:

Your local farm store (check there first!)

Gardener's Supply Company

http://www.gardeners.com

Lehman's Hardware

http://www.lehmans.com

Lady Farmer

http://www.lady-farmer.com

Carhartt Workwear

http://www.carhartt.com

WEBSITES YOU MIGHT ENJOY:

A Farm Girl in the Making

http://www.afarmgirlinthemaking.com

Timber Creek Farm

http://www.timbercreekfarmer.com

Reformation Acres

http://www.reformationacres.com

The Nerdy Farm Wife

http://www.thenerdyfarmwife.com

SCIENTIFIC EVIDENCE RESOURCES:

World Health Organization
   http://www.who.int/en/
PubMed
   http://www.ncbi.nlm.nih.gov/pubmed
Journal of Animal Science and Biotechnology
   https://jasbsci.biomedcentral.com/
University of Maryland Medical Center
   http://www.umm.edu

Index

187; plantain aloe, 189; recipes, 186–90; shea butter, 188

soil, 54–60; fertilizer and, 60; mulch and, 57–58; no-tilling method, 58–59; ph level, 54–55; rich, 55–60; tilling, 57–59

Solanaceae family, cayenne (capsicum), 24

spice mix, herb, 207

spicy eggs, bacon, and kale, 210–11

spinach quiche, 217–19

sprain salve, 155–56

St. John's wort, 47–48

standard rosemary, 45–46

standard yarrow, 51–52

starting herbs, 69–76

Stellaria media, 89

stinging nettle, 85–86

storing herbs, 101–03, 107–08; dried, 107–08

sunlight: drying herbs in, 106; seeds and, 71

supplies, 292–93; livestock, 294

sweet basil, 21

sweet bay, 22

switchel, honey ginger, 231–32

Symphytum spp., 27–28

syrups, 291; basic, 131–32; cough, 133; elderberry, 126, 127–29; flavored, 129–32; ginger honey, 134; honey, 126, 132–34; livestock, 293; medicinal, 125; shelf life, 126

Taraxacom officinale, 84–85

tea, herbal, 110, 111–12, 292; chai latte, 232–33; making, 114–15; mixes, 113; poultry waterer, 282–87; sleep-encouraging, 115; types, 114–16; winter warming, 285–86

tea tree: dog and 276–77; dusting spray, 245; honey, dog, 276–77

thyme, 48–50, 79, 147

thyme biscuits, 224–25

Thymus vulgaris, 48–50

tilling soil, 57–59

tincture(s), 110, 122; alcohol, 119; antibacterial, 266–67; antiviral, 266–67; deworming dog, 277–79; dosage, 118–20, 265; folk method, 123–24; glycerite, 119; herbal, 117–23; liquids, 118–19; livestock, 264–67, 293; parasite,

264–65; poultry antiviral, 286–87; preparing, 120–23; ratio, 119–20; recipes, 120–23; safety, 118; worming, 265–66

toilet spray, 176–77

tonic, herb, 4–6, 67

tooth powder, peppermint, 178

transplanting plants, 74–75

Trifolium pretense, 88–89

true bay, 22

true lavender, 35–36

turmeric, 50–51

turmeric pickles, 222–23

udder balm, livestock, 268

udder wash, livestock, 268–69

urinary tract infection, dog, 277–78

Urtica dioica, 85–86

Urticaceae family, stinging nettle, 85–86

vegetables, herbs and, 65–66

Verbascum spp., 92–93

verdolaga, 93–94

vertical gardening, 64

vinaigrette, herb, 228

Viola odorata, 90

Violaceae family, wild violet, 90

water, seeds and, 71

wild cherry bark, 122

wild herbs, 81–109

wild marjoram, 40–41

wild violet, 90, 130–31; syrup, 130–31

wild violet syrup, simple, 130–31

window cleaner, 243

winterizing herbs, 76–78

wormwood, 247

yarrow, 51–52, 94, 147

yellow ginger, 50–51

Young's dosage rule, 9

Zingiber officinale, 34–35

Zingiberaceae family: ginger, 34–35; turmeric, 50–51